SELF DEFENSE

What You Need to Know to Survive an Attack on the Street or in Your Home

(How to Protect Yourself With the React Self Defence System and Personal Safety)

Grant L Roberts

Published by Bengion Cosalas

Grant L Roberts

All Rights Reserved

ISBN 978-1-77485-351-1

Legal & Disclaimer

The information contained in this book is not designed to replace or take the place of any form of medicine or professional medical advice. The information in this book has been provided for educational and entertainment purposes only.

The information contained in this book has been compiled from sources deemed reliable, and it is accurate to the best of the Author's knowledge; however, the Author cannot guarantee its accuracy and validity and cannot be held liable for any errors or omissions. Changes are periodically made to this book. You must consult your doctor or get professional medical advice before using any of the suggested remedies, techniques, or information in this book.

TABLE OF CONTENTS

Introduction

This book outlines the most effective steps and strategies for using efficient and practical martial arts strategies to defend yourself or your family members. Self-defense is an essential human right. It's also a vital capability that will help you for the rest of your life.

It is not feasible for everyone to invest months or years learning various self-defense techniques. In addition there are many aspects of martial arts can be used for self-defense. That's the purpose on this publication: to assist people of all ages to use simple practical, efficient, and effective martial arts strategies and techniques which can be utilized in real-world situations. This book also offers suggestions on how to stay secure on the streets.

Chapter 1: Train Your Brain To Think Fast!

Each issue we have to face in our lives begins with the mind. If you are able to control your thoughts in any battle, you've already won half the fight. For those who are beaten by a tyrant, their most likely to be a victim of their size or absence of muscle, but the speed in their minds!

If someone freezes when confronted with the opposition, they might be kicked, punched, and even bitten multiple times before even noticing the situation. In the end, knowledge is power, and the ability to anticipate the actions of your opponent in real-time is an enormous game changer. To be able to put together an effective defense, you must master the art of thinking quickly!

Honing Your Reflexes

Reflexes - you either have them or not do you? Wrong! Reflexes are an integral part of an acquired process. Reacting quickly to obstacles that come in is a fundamental aspect of survival.

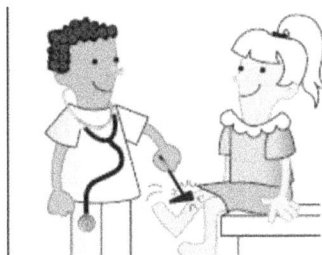

The more often you utilize it, the stronger your reflexes will get. But for most people, it's not easy to develop this skill naturally. It's not impossible, with the exception of rush hour traffic -- it's not every day that we are required to run, jump or dodge obstacles like our lives was on the line.

Our ancestors of the distant past had many physical challenges that honed their reflexes on a regular basis. Think of the hunter-gatherer caveman of 10,000 years ago , who was navigating the forest to chase after wild animals. He was jumping over the roots, squeezing under branches , and throwing spears at swiftly moving wooly mammals simultaneously.

He was taught how to react to events coming at him in just less than a second. A pretty intense method of sharpening your reflexes, don't you think? This is the same in self-defense and fighting. If someone is involved in numerous fights, they'll eventually be able to duck, block and hold on to the punches that fly at them.

It's just natural. As with everything other thing in the world, you'll only be hit a few times before the clever self-defense mechanisms of your body devise a strategy to stay clear of it. It does this by using reflexes. With that being said, the majority of us wouldn't like to get involved engaged in fights for quicker reaction times!

What else should we be doing? There are couple of methods of getting those reactions flowing, without getting into bars on a regular basis. All you need to do is participate in activities that force you to require quick reactions. Skateboarding, for example, could fall into this category.

Skateboarding is a sport where you need to swiftly change direction, adjust and dodge - this is great for developing reflexes. It's as silly as it sounds one of the best options is to play dodge ball.

If you're able to locate an active participant (who wouldn't love playing dodgeball?) Simply ask them to throw an object at you, so that you have to be alert to stay clear of it. This increases blood flow and your reaction speed is enhanced.

The most effective method, which brings us back to the earlier cavemen's story who lived 10,000 years ago--is to run through a forest area that has dense overgrowth. Instead of slowing down to navigate the rough terrain, you should run at a high speed, so that you have to make quick decisions to avoid being struck by branches.

This will make you be able to think quickly to stay safe from being struck by tree branches. Imagine that someone is following you, then race as if your life was on the line from one side in the woods to next.

It is possible to develop excellent scratches in the beginning and also smell like bug repellant (tick time can get quite terrible) But after doing the same thing several times, your reflexes will become improved. With a refined arsenal of reflexes, are able to defend yourself almost second nature to you.

Learn to think on your Feet

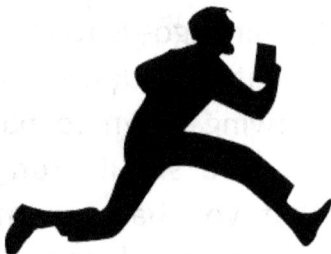

To survive the mind has to be well-equipped. You must be able to process information in the moment they are presented to you. If , for instance, you are confronted with a knife in your throat on the subway, you have to to decide quickly the best option is.

Do you need to run? Do you scream? Do you need to remove the knife out of the attacker's hand? In such circumstances, you must think -- and think quickly. There are several methods to increase the speed of processing in your mind in this respect. Certain involve exercising and physical activity; others could involve enhancing the abilities of our minds.

Here are some great examples:

Do Aerobics!

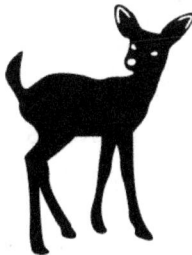

Aerobics can stimulate blood circulation and the breathing flowing! It's also great for helping to concentrate your mind on the goal of self-defense and survival. Aerobics is a physical workout that helps you become familiar with the body's systems and organs and how they function. This understanding allows for more efficient processing speed when applying all these multitasking abilities to work.

Participate in Speed Reading

If your mind were like a pencil, and speed reading was an exercise in sharpening your pencil. There's something in being able to read over the words on an article that naturally boosts the processing capacity of your mind. Words are inextricably linked to our brains' functions and when our language centers are energized by the simple act of the process of reading, our processing speed begins to go to the top!

Utilize Concentrated Meditation

Sometimes, it's not how you act, it's what you aren't doing. Many people meditate as the process of putting the brain into "Safe Mode". As the computer which has to reprocess some items while in Safe Mode, when we do our meditation, we're capable of clearing out lots of things isn't needed. Meditation relieves our minds from many burdens. As consequently, when you restart, you'll notice that your processing speed is improved and you'll be able to think on your feet!

Make sure you are taking your vitamins

Sometimes, if you feel a little sluggish, it could be because the body is not getting enough nutrients. There are a variety of vitamins available available to enhance our cognitive performance. If you think you require an additional boost, you are welcome to give them a try.

Chew gum

A lot of people are surprised by that the simple act of chewing gum could actually boost your brain's power. This is due to the fact that chewing gum increases blood flow to the brain. This in turn providing your brain with greater nutrients for the tasks you're working on. See! I was sure I wasn't sitting with a chewing gum jar at my desk to get something for nothing!

Be on the lookout for

Being aware of dangers prior to it ever happening can give you an enormous advantage should you be defending yourself against threats. There are five senses to be aware of to protect ourselves and we must use them. That means keeping your eyes on the lookout for any unusual activity and keeping your ears open to any hostility that may be lingering.

Let's take, for instance an individual who is in night, and is hanging out at an incredibly busy nightclub on the weekend. The club is bustling and patrons are all over. There's nothing unusual about that is it?

However, you observe from an angle of eyes someone in particular who is constantly watching you. You don't need to be worried however, such an incident will alert you that there's a possible danger in the surrounding. If you notice this quickly enough, you should take action to address it. This doesn't necessarily mean engaging with the person or having a conversation with them.

It's just a matter of being vigilant by watching your back, and trying to stay clear of them, if you can. There are five senses that provide reasons and must adhere to these. To stay safe you must be vigilant at all times. Similar to a deer the forest, which is open to potential hunters, in the wild forest of life , you must be sure to keep an eye on the ground.

Chapter 2: Hand To Hand Self-Defense

The methods below for hand-to-hand self-defense are built on The Krav maga, a form of hand-to-hand combat developed in The Israeli Defense Forces and features heavy emphasis on straightforward and practical strategies. One of the main components of Krav maga revolves on hitting the body's soft spots as the main method of any effective response. The primary focus is on the groin, throat, ears, knees jaw, eyes, nose, as well as Achilles tendon. These body parts are unable to be strengthened through traditional methods that, in turn, creates them as very effective targets, regardless of the person who is your adversary or the level of training they've received.

If you are practicing the techniques described in the next pages it is recommended you do it with the assistance of a friend in a wide, clear space. It is also important to begin slowly and be cautious as it is possible to hurt someone you're training with once you have come to grips with the complete effectiveness of each move. It is best to add speed when you feel at ease with every move, while practicing it with precision. For those who don't have any other partner or a punching bag that is heavy, it could be a good stand-in.

Form a fist in the right way: Perhaps it is not so surprising that the key to successful hand-to-hand self-defense lies in knowing how to construct the correct fist. For a proper fist it is necessary to be bending your fingers to their base , then curl your results into the fist. Don't put your thumb directly on the fist or finish with the fingers touching because this can be a great method of breaking it if things become physically.

If you are using a closed hand to attack another person the goal should be to strike the most affluent knuckles that are located on your pointer and middle fingers. They will create more forceful impact, which can result in more damage to the victim's soft tissues. When you are throwing a punch, you'll need to stand with your feet flat and then move them from the hip to produce the maximum potent strike force.

Focus on the groin area: If the person you are fighting is male, there's no more efficient or faster method of destroying them than with a swift and powerful blow into the groin. To get the most benefit from this strike you will be required to start with what is called a staggered stance by sitting with the dominant foot in front of your second leg. Then, you'll need to make use of your hip flexors and your quads to push straight forward , then up. While doing this you will need to slightly lean back towards your waist in order to keep your equilibrium. If you are using this technique you will need to try to bring your shin directly with the muscles of your attacker's groin.

While films may teach us to aim for the kick with our knees or even the foot however, in actual combat this approach is not always practical. The shin benefits of being both easy to target because of its greater surface area, and also providing the most force from your body. When you are preparing on the strike, you shouldn't just rest at your groin area, imagine kicking upwards through your body to ensure that you are able to follow through enough to be able to count the punch.

Refuse to take a hit from the outside. This is a fundamental defensive technique that can help to defend yourself against attacks, slaps and punches as well as blunt weaponry directed at your face. Training this technique every day is vital to your overall success combat because it will ensure that your body is properly reacted to in the event of being struck. Absolutely, getting hit with your arm is significantly less painful than being struck in the arm.

In order to perform this action for this move, you'll be able to lift your arms out and up to shield your face as the attacker comes in to ensure that your fingers point towards the upward direction as well as your elbow bent slightly. If the attacker begins to strike, you are going to be lifting your forearm until it is moving upwards to the inside of the attacker's arm. While doing this you'll be able to utilize the deflecting arm to raise your other arm into the perfect position to strike at the jaw, throat or nose , based on where you can reach easily at when you are at the point. The arm that performs the deflection will differ based on the arm is being used by the attacker for the strike.

Escape when you are grabbed by the back: This technique is perfect when an attacker is able to grab you from behind and hold your arms to your sides. For starters, you're likely to bring your weight quickly, as like you're doing the Squat. The goal is to lower the center of gravity of your body, making it harder for the attacker to move or lift your body. To begin, you're likely to need to position your feet in a position where they are higher than the hip width. After that, you'll be able to shift your hips away from the sides so that you are able to move backwards with your dominant hand to grab the area of your groin.

Once the path is cleared, you're likely be able to keep your hand in the open position and strike them with maximum force in the hope of releasing their grip. If the grip is loosening it is then time to move forward as far as you can in order to gain the advantage before ramming your arm into the stomach of your attacker before turning back to confront them in one seamless move. This should give you the freedom to add more punches that target the body's natural weak points , or to run when the situation calls for.

Get rid of a backwards strangulation attempt: In lieu of giving you an embrace the attacker goes straight towards your throat and attempts to block the airway in your throat, it is essential not to go fighting in vain, since you will only have the time to react with enough force to create a change. This technique will require more time than the other because the body is conditioned to respond negatively to an extended lack of air.

The best option in this scenario is to step into a staggered stance prior to lifting the arm close to the forward-facing staggered leg. It is best to raise the arm straight until your bicep is close to the ears. Then, you'll want to cross your leg that is facing forward in front of your rear leg and then turn back to the direction that the leg was crossing, rotating toward your elevated arm while doing so. While doing this you will need to be aggressive and as fast as you can throw your bodyweight and all the force you can get to your opponent's wrists.

Then you should be facing your attacker , and completely free of their grasp which allows you to run or fight depending on the circumstances. If executed correctly, the move will cause the attacker to stumble and put them in a position that you are able to respond with multiple blows at their weak points.

Take off a one-handed choke on a wall: This is a good option when you are being pinned against a wall while holding one hand firmly around your throat. If someone is putting you in a choke to the wall typically, they will make you do what they want for you to comply with. So, the very first thing you're going to be tempted to do is move around to give the impression that you are following their instructions. This should make them lower their guards enough for you to make your first step, and then be sure to make it count.

For the first step, you're likely to want to pull your chin into your chest, pressing on the thumb of your attacker to break their grip when you do this. Once you have done this, you'll then need you to lift your arms, with your palms fully open, right next to the wrist that your adversary is using in order to grip your body on the walls. It is then important to use the hand that isn't your dominant hand to grasp the wrist that is in question and then drive it to the ground making use of your hand that is dominant to create a an ideal fist and strike the weak spots of the attacker's face. To ensure that your punch is as effective as you can move your hips around while striking to give your punch an additional amount of force. After that, you can knee to your groin to move your attacker backward and allow yourself to move.

If you need to disarm someone holding the knife to your throat If you're in a situation in which an attacker is armed and holding an instrument in your throat, from behind. The best step to take is not be in a get scared. Any uncontrolled movement can cause possibly life-threatening injuries, therefore it is crucial to make sure you are careful and controlled in your actions.

To begin, you'll want to appear as if you're going to comply with the wishes of your attacker in order in order to force them to release their grip. Then, using a quick controlled motion , you're going to be able to place your hands together on the wrists of the person who holds the knife. Then as you hold it to your chest, push down with all the strength you can. Keep going with the bulk of your weight in the process, pulling your chin back to ensure that you're looking towards the knife.

Following this step will assist in shifting the knife's threat away from the most vulnerable parts, making the attack less risky. When the knife is away from your face, you're likely to need to use your hand that isn't in the position of holding the knife to hit the stomach. When they're out of balance, you're then likely to use the arm close to your arm sitting on your chest. You will then place your head in their armpit, while maintaining your chin down and their wrists secure. You will then need you to turn your legs in the direction of shifting your body so that you're in the direction of the person who is attacking you instead of facing them in the forward. Then, you'll want to continue this action with the foot that is closest to the attacker's to drop the entire force onto their foot , causing them to fall off balance and then shoving them into the ground.

Chapter 3: How to Get Away

Synopsis

Self-protection doesn't just mean understanding a few tricks It's all about the actions we take every day to improve our lives. A lot of this is common sense, and the rest simply adds to. There are some things that you can perform without thinking about whether it's wearing a belt and crossing the road, or operating a knife with care. When people used to be forced to wear seatbelts inside the car, now people are able to sit in their cars and open their arms without thought. This shows that when you repeat something repeatedly that it becomes an habit and eventually it becomes automatic.

Escape

The way you look at the ground, lowering your shoulders, putting your hands in pockets, and making yourself appear small conveys the message "I'm weak and vulnerable". Women are viewed as easy targets and using a firm posture reduces the likelihood of being fair in the game.

Engage with others in a way that they can see that you've observed the person (wishful criminals are much less likely to commit a crime in the event that they fear they will be identified). Move your arms as you walk or soaking up the air. Your body language is not just is about how people perceive you, but also increases your confidence in yourself.

Make a comparison of street-based enemies with wild animals They're not looking for the largest, most bold and most invulnerable animal to attack, but rather the fragile, wounded or sever. Do not put yourself in a place that increases your vulnerability. Predators don't want to fight but rather a simple kill. If the person in the position is fighting hard, the predator is likely to abort.

Self-confidence is an essential element of gaining control over your life. If the conduct of someone else makes you feel uncomfortable, uneasy or anxious, then speak up to them. Inform them of the behavior, critique it, then tell them what you'd like them to do "You're always touching me and I'm not happy about the way you're doing it, get rid of it" Repeat the statement if needed. This is a clear method of communicating your goals; you should avoid making a statement of "please" while affirming yourself. If someone is causing you trouble in public places and you are angry, then go on the offensive. It is more humiliating for the person who is causing the problem than for you. Your voice is also a weapon.

Your hollering could alert others about and may alarm an attacker. It can also help channel your terror into aggression. Scream "NO" loudly and deeply in your abdomen. Follow your instincts. If there's a problem with something or appear to be in the right place, it probably isn't. If you suspect that someone has been in your vicinity - trust your gut and take action such as approaching them, bringing them to the safety zone, calling someone or making a weapon.

Consider a mobile phone, it's cheap when it's used for emergency purposes it is not just a way to gather help from anywhere, but you can make use of it to carry out a range of tasks.

Make sure to use your voice when an encounter that is forcible has begun. The loud screams you make when you attack can serve multiple purposes. In the first place, you may make the attacker frightened by the sound of a scream that is loud and sudden, you're making yourself visible so that someone can come to help you or help you. Additionally, you could have witnesses that could prove useful in the event that you caused physical injury to your attacker.

to defend yourself, you could be a situation in which it's one of your words against another's but if it occurred that a passing motorist was able to hear you shouting "Let go let it go" and that is now evidence. Shouting can also increase the size of your abdominal muscles, which means that if you receive a blow at the at the same time, you're less likely to get out of breath due to it.

It is logical that the closer to your attacker, the shorter time you will have to react to their movements. In other words, the more distance between you and your attacker, the longer time you'll need to respond.

Maintain a safe distance, one that is comfortable for you and gives you enough time to respond. If you can, stand with the obstruction in that is between your and another person as well.

The attacker always has the advantage from an action reaction perspective since he's aware of the fact that he's going out but your brain needs to analyze what you're doing and decide what you're likely to do to react and then transmit the signals to the muscles so that they move in the manner necessary.

Chapter 4: The Rise of Violence The Rise

In our modern society violence is the only thing that is unavoidable, regardless of gender, age or the social status evident in our daily lives. Statistics from around the world show that every two minutes an individual woman is victimized or sexually assaulted by an uninvolved person. 30 percent or more of children in North America experience being bullied in one way or another. The number of crimes is on the rise in a number of countries. The list continues across the globe.

Such reports can cause us to enter an anxious state of mind and stress , imagining that something similar can happen to us once we leave our home. The worst part is that it could occur right the doorway of our step. While local police officers are mandated to safeguard the population, it's the responsibility of each individual to safeguard themselves in circumstances arise.

How To Handle It

To safeguard oneself from being attacked, learning self-defense is encouraged by people who are concerned about the issue. Many people believe that by taking self-defense classes, acts of criminality can be prevented and also be used as a warning for those who wish to harm someone else.

Self-defense training does not always need to be reserved for healthy and fit female or male. It can be taught to older adults who are physically fit. Particularly for those living on their own or do not have a family member to count on when confronted by a crisis.

How to Improve Self-Defense

There are many methods to improve your self-defense skills and safeguard yourself from the people who would like to harm you. You can join the martial arts academy. If you have a buddy who is experienced, who can guide you through the fundamentals of self-defense. Organise your neighborhood and ask your local authority for police to establish an education program on self-defense. The main objective is to train yourself aware of what to do in the event of the threat of violence.

How do you overcome Fear

The majority of us prefer to think that we're incapable of defending ourselves by ourselves due to our weaknesses or fears. You'll be amazed at how simple it is to overcome this feeling once you've begun to master the fundamentals of self-defense. As time passes your confidence will begin to grow and will eventually take over the task of removing your anxiety and stress. The benefits are to both your mental and physical health.

Self Defense without Physical Confrontation

Self-defense doesn't have to mean facing an attacker physically but it can also be achieved by being street-wise. For instance , if you believe that you're being stalkedby someone, don't go in a direction in which you'll be alone. Always follow the route where you'll be surrounded numerous people until you are able to seek assistance. Another option is to learn how to talk when confronted by an adversary. Sometimes, it's better to surrender your power instead of remorseting the result.

While self-defense training cannot completely assure us that we'll be able to get away from a potential attack without sustaining any physical injuries but it certainly increases the chance of survival or deterring the attacker from attacking us.

Chapter 5: The Throw

Throwing is the primary move in grappling. If executed correctly, it will turn the battle to your advantage by providing you with a advantage in position. But to execute it, you need some ability. It is generally required to step back and stutter your opponent before throwing him. For beginners, however you could practice throwing by having a steady partner as you try throwing him. Strikes and other tumbling movements will be addressed in a subsequent chapter.

As with grips, there's no one perfect throw you can throw at your opponent. It's going to be based on a variety of factors, including location, size, and strength. When you read this chapter, I would suggest you and a buddy test the techniques in a secure area like a gym or a place in which mats or padding is accessible. It is only through experience that you can decide which throws are suitable for you.

In the subsequent throws it is assumed you already have your opponent's hand.

Major Outer Reaping Throw. This throw can be a powerful move when you have an upper hand on the clothing of your opponent. To throw it, you must make use of the dominant leg to one side opposite to your opponent from their back to his (your rear). This will knock your opponent's balance and cause them to sink to the ground.

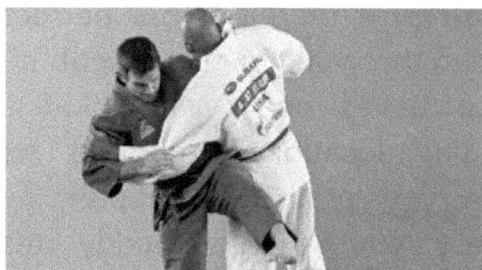

The Major Outer Reaping Throw. Image obtained by Blackbelt (n.d.).

There's a variant of this throwing. As you first grasped your opponent's clothes the hands of your opponent should be easily released. If you are sweeping the leg of your opponent, grab him by the chin and then throw at him with the intention that he is falling. This will accelerate his fall and significantly slam him.

Hip Throw. If you're physically strong, this throw will be extremely damaging to your opponent when he's heavy or wearing an obstructive clothing. To do it, take your opponent's balance and bring him towards his right front by pulling his back. Also swiftly turn your back to ensure that both of you face the in the same direction. Make use of his loss of balance to quickly volley your opponent with your hips. While doing this, ensure that your knees are bent to the point that your opponent is able to slide over you. This will give you the stability and strength. You'll know you've done the correct way when you feel your opponent's groin pressing against your lower part.

The hip Throw. Image was taken by Tony On Jiu Jitsu (2014).

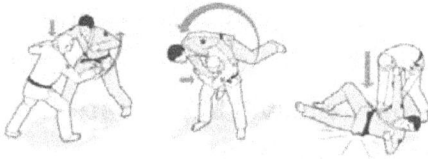

The Major Internal Reaping Throw. This throw is ideal for those who want to get over your opponent, and then transition into a succession of swift punches. To do this, you must break the balance of your opponent by using your left leg in order to force his left leg ahead. Then, he will fall backwards. In order to get your right foot into the legs of your opponent it is necessary to make the sweep motion. This motion of sweeping will enable you to effectively knock over your opponent. If your opponent falls, you don't have to fall, in the event that you lose your balance. This is an excellent chance to get away. Or, you can slide over your opponent to ensure that you are able to be able to subdue him.

The Major Reaping Inner Throw. Image obtained by Pinterest (n.d.).

Shoulder Throw. Shoulder throws are identical to that of the Hip Throw, only with more force since you're moving your opponent with your shoulder instead of using your hips. To do this, you must break the opponent's balance by lifting his face towards yours. While you're doing this, you should move your right foot in the direction of the opponent's. Make sure to turn your back as long as your opponent remains standing and bend your knees and then use each hand to throw the opponent across your shoulder. You may find you can use your elbow to provide leverage against the armpit of your opponent will let you throw him more easily across your own body.

The Shoulder Throw. Image obtained from Judo Channel (n.d.).

KO-UCHI-GARI

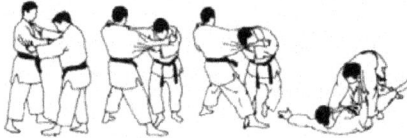

Minor Reaping of the Ankle. This throw is identical to the major inner reaping throw, however this throw is focused to throw your adversary sideways back and not towards the back of his direct. This is a straightforward throw you can make to easily gain a advantage in position over your opponent. You can make your opponent unstable to the right side as you use your left step to sweep the left side toward his front. After you've done this your opponent will appear unbalanced, but he will not slide. This is a great opportunity to force your opponent to the side. To make yourself more secure You may discover that headbutting becomes more efficient.

The Minor Outer Reaping Throw. Image was taken in Judo Info (n.d.).

A Sweeping Ankle Throw. It is a basic but deadly throw that will totally confuse your opponent if that you are strong enough. To accomplish this, put your right foot in front of you. This will make your opponent think that you are move backwards with the left side of his foot. Make a left-hand step. Make sure that your left leg is strong enough to support your weight. If your opponent's weight remains on his left foot swiftly move his left ankle to sweep it as you pull him towards his upper left. It will make sure that the opponent remains sitting on the ground. Make sure to move quickly since your opponent has plenty of time to react, and stop the right side of your leg moving towards him.

A Sweeping Ankle Throw. Photograph is taken via Memrise (n.d.).

The Body Drop Throw. This throw is a great way to strike your opponent's body a bit further from your body compared to the throws above. This gives you plenty of time to adjust your posture or simply get away. For this, take your opponent off balance by lifting him to the right front. This will cause him to lose the foundation of your left foot. Make sure that your right foot is blocking his right ankle as well as the left leg is bent slightly. When your opponent is raised, swiftly rotate him and throw your opponent in the direction of forward. Straighten your legs so you'll have more energy when you throw your opponent. You'll know that you did it right if the opponent's body is not directly in front of you.

The Body Drop Throw. Image was taken by Return of Kings (2016).

The Sweeping Hip Throw. This throw is an amalgamation with throwing the Hip

Throw and the Sweeping Ankle Throw. The throw will knock your opponent off of his equilibrium by pulling him to his right side. When you're doing this, place with your right foot to the right of your opponent's foot. With your left leg fixed to the ground, turn your body in a backward direction to ensure that both of you look in the in the same direction. While doing this, hold your opponent's waist or neck. Utilize your left leg for pushing against the left side of their opponent. This will lift away your adversary from the ground. Use your arms quickly to push your foe in the direction of forward.

It is the Sweeping Hip Throw. Image obtained from Judo Channel (n.d.).

Intimate Thigh Throw. This throw is best suited to those who aren't skilled enough to throw precisely, but who have good balance. To make this throw take you balance by bringing your opponent by moving his front right. Move your right foot toward the opponent's. Your left foot must serve as your anchor. Then, turn your body around and place your right arm on the waist or neck that of your adversary. Utilize your right thigh to sweep upwards and then backwards to raise your opponent's legs. Your right thigh should follow your left leg of your opponent , so that you can throw him in the right way. When you are ready, quickly and forcefully throw your opponent straight to the front.

The Inner Thigh Throw. Image is taken via JudoInfo (n.d.).

Fireman's Lift. The Fireman's Lift is ideal for those who are in an awkward position due to being sitting on the floor. The lift requires you to stand kneeling with one leg. For this, you must position yourself so that you're kneeling with one leg bent and the other kneeling. It is also possible to move your knees. Utilize your right arm to grasp your opponent's body with the thigh's back. Then, move your feet toward to the center of his legs. Utilize your right hand hold your opponent's sleeves. Then pull the sleeves down so that your opponent's back will rest on your shoulders.

Chapter 6: Self Defense For Woman - Fight To Survive An Attack

In the event that you ever have a moment when you must fight for your life, I suggest you don't hesitate. Take on the enemy. It can save your life. Many physical assaults have been rebuffed because of how the victims was fighting with the attacker. Studies show that the woman who fights has a better chance of surviving and getting away than the woman who does not aid the fight. In the event that an individual is attempting to harm you or your family, he's out to hurt you regardless of the circumstances. Engaging him in combat will make him feel awestruck and because the attacker must escape with a little resistance most of the time, he'll allow your rights to get away from him. An attacker isn't a fan of an excessive amount of noise So, make a significant amount. You should holler as long and as hard that you are able to. Make statements that draw into your mind.

"HELP I'm being attacked by him!" "HELP! He's ATTACKING ME! "I do not have any contact with HIM I'm not even a friend with him! HE'S Endeavoring TO Seize ME! Someone is trying to help me" - "CALL the Police, he's Harming Me!" "HELP me this MAN is following me!"

Okuri-Ashi-Barai

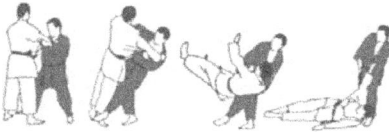

If you're in a public space and you suspect that someone is following or following you. Look at his face. Make sure he is aware that you can see him. Speak loudly "I See you. Let me sit in peace now." "POLICE!! POLICE!!" He'll ponder bounces at the police. In the event that you're separated from all the other people and you sense that someone is watching you, avoid being snatched up. Go to a place that is open such as a public area with close people or the man. If you are in danger, you are in need of help, you can ask for someone to accompany you to your vehicle or get ready to take the group and aid. This could also mean that you are defenceless on your own or being protected by the assistance of another group.

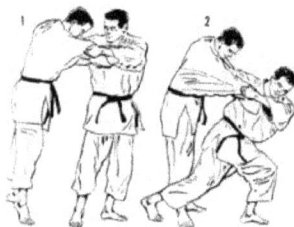

These are just a few of the strategies to avoid attacks. It may seem obvious, but they are meant to be a to refer to. Beware of going to dim locations without any other people in the event that you're able. Take a walk with a friend whenever you are able. In the event that there's a bright spot or a lamp, stay in the vicinity. Keep away from someone who is trying to corner you or to group you up but don't go towards a spot that may be more hazardous for you. As an example, don't get closer towards the track of an plan in the event that you don't know the things this person could be capable of. Know who's close to you and the number of people are in the vicinity. Know who is around and the way they dress. Be aware of any erratic behavior such as hostility, alcoholism or a shrewd behavior. Be aware of relationships regardless of whether or not a person isn't in a relationship with someone doesn't mean that they're not part of a group. There will be signs of connection when that you sit for a long time. You'll see connections is trying to hide or conceal. You will also see indications of each other's glances. However when something starts to happen the pair will make their involvement public. They'll come after you as a couple. Don't believe that because you are seeing a woman in a relationship with a male that they're not a threat to you. Usually, women are attracted to you

47

and when you take down your defenses and later, for various reasons, mostly for the part, to please the man who they are with, you offer the man the chance to confront you, or they are likely to attack each other. There are many Bonnie and Clyde writes out on the internet. Just be aware of partnerships.

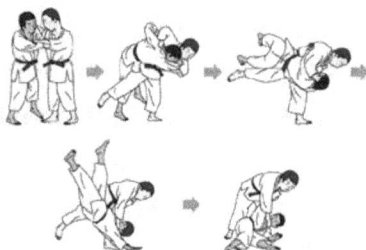

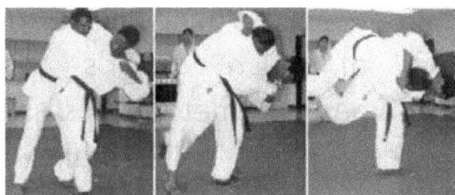

A few suggestions: Don't open your purse when you are out in public. Make sure to set up your keys or cash prior to leaving a location. Transfer a key securely between your two fingers , and your thumb, with the pointed end visible. In the event that you're being snatched away, don't run randomly. Before you head out on any route, be aware of whether it is an escape route or deadlock. When walking, you must be aware about the nature. The entrances that people can hide with, paths or passageways that are shrouded in mystery, as well as typical landmasses that may hinder your from being a hiding spot for someone. Be aware of areas where there are people who can assist you. Are there any corner stores that are open late? restaurants, fire stations and Police headquarters. Find out about call boxes and really check to see if they're working or not. If you need to make the telephone to call, you should be aware of historical aspects to offer some fantastic tips. If you are carrying a bag that is not a purse, it's better for you to choose a bag that is divided into compartments and you usually put your items in the bag in the same place. When you're in need of your wallet, phone or lipstick, you are able to retrieve it using the flickering of your eyes or not even a glance or imagination. A person who is calm has a lower chance of being focused or in check as compared to a complex person. An individual who is focused and focused is also more likely to become a victim or an objective person than someone who is solitary and distracted. Walk with a sense of purpose and believe that you do not know where you're traveling. Plan your courses for your residence, your school, or a store, and so on. Additionally, there are optional safe courses that are prepared to change courses in just a few minutes should the need arises. If you are aware of a few ways to get to a place, you'll be able to take a decisive step and not swerve.

If you're attacked, be set to fight until there is no quality to offer your self, or until the person is completely unaware. There are three main areas in which a person is defenceless: his crotch; his eyes, and his knees. If someone is trying to attack you, kick, punch and kick, knee strike, get, crush or strike at him or even bite the genitals of him until the point where you are able to be free. In the event that the person falls to his knees due to the blow, punch him with your eyes or take the rear of your head and strike him with a knee or clench your hands using two hands, and then place them onto his head as forcefully as you can to the point where he goes to the ground. Punch him or kick him repeatedly over and over in the crotch area. In the event that you are chasing his eyes, try to pull them away, or put your fingers and hands together like a feathered nose and strike your fingers and hands hard at him. Be prepared that he may strike you with his hands clenched or a hand that is accessible.

Make yourself ready for any hits or strikes that he might throw at you. Whatever happens you don't put it off because your life is in the in the balance! If he is attempting to strike your face or head by using something similar to an axe, a stick or even a tough question, secure your head with your arms and hands. Keep your arms moving as your head to not to cause harm to your face and head. It's better to take strikes on your arm rather than to your head or face. Hit him with your feet , or put him on the knees when he's threatening you. If you are unable to reach his crotch, strike his knee by using the sole of your feet. Keep on kicking him until you reach the point where he releases you. If you are thumps then twist your legs towards your body, and hold your arms straight and your hands in front of you to secure both your face and the head. Look at your goal and then really kick your feet and into some of his knees difficult as you can in the event you are able to reach the crotch of his. Don't bother trying to get the head or face of your opponent or face, he might get your feet or legs injured when you strike his face. Strike hard or forcefully at his crotch, knees and eyes. If you do cut him Don't stop there take the initiative to attack. Keep him moving using the feet initially. Wrap his head around or around his crotch, and use your feet to sledges, or a hatchet. Slash downwards with your back area to his head or crotch repeatedly where he's exposed. Do the same to him with your hands. Do not think that as he's down you can't help him up again. Don't think after you kicked him in his crotch , he will not have the strength to rise again. He could be angry enough that it is able to divert his attention from the pain and pursues you. Therefore, keep going until the attacker stops, or is not paying attention, or you are able to break off and seek help.

Even though you're not carrying a weapon, you're not at risk. Take everything you're carrying as a possible device or weapon. You could be able to lure him into a trap. In fact, even the most sluggish daily paper or magazine could be on the way towards being something more substantial when used correctly. The final page of a rolled up newspaper or magazine could be smacked into the crotch area of his. The bag can also be smashed through his bottom. The wooden handle of an umbrella could cause pain if slammed into the crotch of his. A stick that is suggestive can be smacked into the eye of a child. Pens or keys could be smacked into his crotch, or into his eye. If you're wearing the high back area or a pair of shoes with a solid rear section put your foot on the instep of your foot. Pummel an object like a book or folder case down his crotch. If the person who lifts you off the ground from behind, yank him up and back into his ribs. Kick your back foot more , then kneel down or kick it up to his hips. You can chomp him while staring at him straight in the face. Use your hands as a an clench and smash your clench hand down and backwards into his crotch area or up and up into the nose of his victim. Use your hands as claws. Make your hand strong in that claw, and throw the hand back downwards into the crotch of his partner as fast as you can. Learn about all the things you are able to use. If you need to restore some calm of a subject that's tough like a stone don't throw it at himas you might miss and not have a second chance with it. Instead, hold it with firmness and when he gets close, take it and smash it against your nose or smack it into the crotch of his. You should hold the stone with the assumption that, after the initial hit, he might be able to see, and he might try to use it against you. Do not provide him with any advantage. You must be ready to employ your weapon or device again until you stop or the weapon transforms into an obstacle instead of providing aid to you.

Whatever happens, if the guy can figure out how to get you on the ground, all is not lost. Be focused on you and your primary interest. He'll anticipate that you'll fight and when you're to the floor, you could imagine you're cooperating. And then, when he aware that you aren't in conflict, he starts to relax and at this point, you release your body of his grasp, fall onto your stomach, pull your legs out of the way, then look around, and take a look at your target and strike him in either his knee or in his crotch. If the man is perched on your head, your chest is pointing towards you and your legs are up, you can swing them upwards to either side and grab him by the chest using your legs. Then, push him backwards with your legs. When he is forced to fall in reverse take him off with your legs and then in a matter of seconds, take the initiative by kicking his crotch or pounding your feet onto his nose or head because he's sitting on the ground, you will find him less tense and more easily reachable. If the person who is bringing you down does try to stay clear of having your situation appear not a good one or getting cuffed but should that occurs, you've got your legs at hand. Take your time and fight with everything you have. Inform him that you are a HERPES or Helper. Anything that can influence him to reconsider. Remember that when you're being targeted by him the consequences are his or yours. The expectation of him is

Chapter 7: Five Basic Self-Defense Techniques

Given the current conditions that we live in there are many good citizens who are being required to commit crimes or hurt others for private, but not legitimate reasons. When you consider the consequences being said, it's important to be aware that we need to be in a position to defend ourselves. With all the expenses piling up within our houses, nobody has time or cash to take classes in self-defense or purchase guns for personal security. In this regard, we have listed the most the most basic self-defense strategies that are easy and simple to master. It's sure to protect you should a specific event occurs.

1. Hit and run

A hit-and-run strategy is ideal and efficient when you're in a circumstance when that is near security, and you're able to escape if you strike or you're in a situation of fear and are in a situation of complete isolation. It's also a useful method if you want to create space between yourself and the attacker prior to when you take out weapons or are prepared to launch a further attack.

Many different techniques of attack are used for hit and run. The key element is footwork. It is essential to be in a place that the attacker can't hurt you , and you'll be able to escape when you are attacked. One of the easiest techniques to master is to use the eye strike.

Eye Strike

* The name basically refers to what you do. Hit the eyes of your adversary by using your fingers.

The stance must be in the shape that of the triangular feet in order to make sure that there is a smooth escape after the strike.

Make sure to bend your knees in the triangular footing. This can greatly reduce the risk of head injuries from the attacker.

When you are attacking the other hand, it should be placed in the side of your back to guard yourself from punches.

2. Blast

The blast is one type of tactic that requires more aggression. Particularly, this method is ideal for situations when you're under threat, or with your loved ones who is unable to escape, and you must get rid of the person who is attacking you.

The blast technique mostly involves continuous high-pressure assaults.

There are a variety of types of attacks are employed.

* In the event of attacks, ensure that you choose the one which best suit your needs and do not forget to cover your head or any vital places.

3. Crash

The crash is an excellent attack against attackers that utilize upper body strikes. This isn't a defense technique but it can be efficient against attackers' hooks, punches, and continual attacks. It is ideal if you are in a position where you're likely to be targeted.

The crash can disrupt the attacker's initial attack, a good example would be to stop an attack.

Let's suppose that the attacker uses the right cross to attack you. Move forward, while blocking the attack by using both of your arms, encasing your face with your arms.

* Make use of your left arm to push the attacker toward your knee, while you right arm should be grabbing the right hand of the attacker.

* When you pull him down, then jam your knee against him. you've destroyed his attack and repelled it by launching your own. Once your attacker has fallen, swiftly flee.

4. Grappling Defense

The grappling defense is a reaction to the tackle, grappling and takedowns that attackers will try to perform. This method does not need to be based on strength or size of the muscle similar to this method that relies upon bone's structure.

* If an attacker attempts to knock you and then you are unable to move, you should back off as soon as you notice him coming.

Be aware that the leg that you use to move back is the one that the attacker's head is turning towards.

When the head is near enough you can make use of your elbow to strike his neck or head.

Note that the arm you utilize to strike should be perpendicular to the direction of your opponent.

5. Clinch Entry

The clinch is a technique to use if you've received an assault and your adversary holds the upper hand. If you're already in the dirt the techniques of crashing and blast will be extremely difficult, or almost impossible to execute.

* If you think you may have been the victim of a beating take a knee and make sure to safeguard your face or head.

You can quickly lunge towards your attacker. It will be similar to hugging him however all your arms must be in his.

* Put him in "the harness" In this way, you will be right behind him.

* Lower him by striking the back of his knee. Secure him in a choke.

If the attacker is gone, you are able to escape.

Chapter 8: Practical Self Defense Strategies For Woman

It's not too late to get started self-defense and the best part is that it doesn't need to be expensive to master! In a matter of minutes, you'll be learning to avoid rape , and how to be able to defend yourself against a simple attack in only 15 minutes!

Practical self-defense strategies We should not steer any attack direction recklessly or rely on contact origins only, however, we must to identify a specific area which is a weak point for man is, so that we are able to defend ourselves regardless of attacks with force or strength that are not seem to be so powerful. Man is a creation of God with a range of weaknesses.

There are weak spots in our bodies which we can exploit in our goal to offer protection when confronted with criminals. The introduction and understanding of these areas are essential even if we have never learned any martial art to make the defense that we offer is truly powerful. Also, keep in mind that since these points are an integral part of the body when it comes to martial arts, and there is no way to in strengthening it.

1. Both Eyes

Eyes are both very vulnerable, as it could cause pain and be blind when it is assaulted. The most common attack on the eyes are the ones that catch our attention by putting one three-quarters of the middle. The the little finger folded over our thumbs. This can with our fingers. This can cause them to become hard. You can also accomplish this with tools like the sand, sharp objects (sticks or pens.) as well as water spray (spray tear gas spray, water chili).

2. Jaw

Jaw is also among the weak spots in the body of a human. The jaw can be attacked in this region by getting striking or punching with a solid object.

3. The Throat

The Throat is an extremely weak spot, as it is a place where pain can go disappear and then return when it is attacked. There are a variety of ways to attack the thrombus are punched using the hand in a half-clenched position. as well as using an object that is pointed (sticks pen, sticks, etc.)

4. Heartburn

Heartburn is a vulnerable area, as it can cause painful and shortness of breath the person who suffers from it if they are struck. One type of attack against heartburn is to attack with your hands half-clenched, or elbows and legs.

5. Public

This point is extremely vulnerable because it could cause the owner feel pain and even hurt the victim if it is it is attacked. The methods of attacking this point include kicking it with your foot or punching.

Chapter 9: Pressure Point Revival

If you are practicing hitting these points, you'll at some point have to revive the part which was hit so that your partner in training will be able to use the body part rapidly. In the acupressure point theory, when you hit a spot, you take energy away. What you must do is bring back the energy that you have lost.

We won't force you to believe that but it's logical that if you hit your trainer or you knock him down it is sensible to learn how you can help him. In this section, we'll go over strategies to assist your trainee to regain physical function.

Take note that if not bring your opponent back to life you will see them awake at some point, but they'll experience discomfort in various parts of their body because of the strikes you applied to different pressure points. It's like waking up with an hangover.

Reviving the Arm

We've pointed out the tension points in the arms. If these points are hit correctly and correctly, you could make your opponent lose their balance or let them slide to ground. They are more likely not to knock someone out, and you can use them to establish other strikes that target other pressure points in the body.

To restore motor function to arms all you have to do is tap the same points on the arm you struck, and afterward, give it a gentle massage. The same spot is hit using your palm open, but only with 50% of the force struck with to strike it. Then, massage the area with your hands. Repeat the procedure if you need to.

Reviving Your Training Partner From the ground

What do you do after the opponent knocks you unconscious? If your opponent is unconscious, it is best to first cross his legs in an upright position. Next, help your training partner sit up. It is best to kneel on his side and with his body in a straight line.

Put one knee against his back (somewhere near the middle or the back of his spine) to stop him from falling down. Keep one hand on the chin to keep his head upright.

The second step would be to pinpoint the spot where you struck the spot, whether on the chest, neck or the. If you hit anywhere in the lower left of your head or neck, it is recommended to revive from the opposite side of the neck or head and reverse.

Then, you will slap the area of the neck where GB 20 is (either either the left, or right, depending on the area you hit). It is home to a nerve in that area known as the wake-up nerve. Repeat the same procedure using the arm strike and slap it at a half force, then massage the region.

This will awake him. The same approach is used when you knocked out your opponent by striking him in either the front or back.

Restore Energy

In order to further aid in restoring consciousness, he may be a little groggy place your forefinger as well as your thumb (not in your palm however, but instead in the side of your hand) on the bottom of the spine of your trainer and then push your hand to the top of his spine with an upward movement. Repeat this three or four more times.

It should suffice to assist your trainer get back to consciousness. He will be back to training within a matter of minutes.

Chapter 10: Responsibility to Retrench - Explained

The obligation to withdraw is a common provision that is found in states' laws on self-defense and recourse to deadly force. The defendants are typically obliged to comply with this clause before the use of the use of deadly force is justifiable. This is required by a few states. In some states, the victim (the person who utilized the force that was deadly) is required to provide showing that the action was reasonable. To be considered reasonable, many states' laws stipulate that the defendant has done whatever was necessary to stop the conflict. The defendant must be able to show that the necessary steps were taken to avoid the danger, and that he did all he could to was not to do to fight, but was forced into resorting to force that was deadly. Certain jurisdictions require that the use of self-defense using deadly force is only justified when the retreat was not feasible or was dangerous for the person being assaulted.

However, this obligation to retreat is not universally recognized. It is contingent on the rules of the state on the matter.

Exclusivity from the obligation to withdraw

A majority of states have took the "no obligation to retreat" policy regarding the violent recourse to force. Around 31 states have adopted this law. A further 19 states have the obligation to withdraw.

The legal systems of many states have begun to adopt English common law, such as those of the Acts of Parliament of 2 Ed. II, or Statute of Northampton and the 5 Rich. II of 1381, also known as the Act for Forcible Entry of 1381. The Forcible Entry Act of 1381. English laws introduced criminal sanctions to discourage citizens from using self-help or force to defend themselves. The law changes obliged the person who was threatened to evade the threat and take every step to settle the issue with civil remedies.

States that have embraced this position prohibit citizens from being able to resort to using deadly force in defense. The jury concludes there was no danger to the person or the grave bodily injury could be avoided had the victim had retreated.

However, this simplifies things. Certain states provide more precise guidelines regarding this provision. For example, the laws of Pennsylvania oblige the need to withdraw when the threatening person (i.e. the attacker) was not carrying a visible weapon that was aimed or poised to cause death or severe physical injury.

The only exceptions to the obligation to retreat include police officers who are they are performing their duty. States that adopt the Castle doctrine will not need anyone to justify the use of using deadly force if the incident occurred within the home. Another instance is when the law of the state has adopted the notion of "stand your the ground".

Chapter 11: Knowing Your Enemy

In the final analysis, they are humans, and they suffer and are swollen like the rest of us. Make sure you target the parts of the body you are most likely to do harm to. This is the neck, face knees, and groin. Take a moment to assess your situation prior to deciding which area to focus you efforts. For instance, don't ever attempt to hit the groin area with a kick , when you can just throw a bag of heavy weight up the nose of him from a further distance.

The face is a great place to strike because it is home to numerous parts that are vulnerable. Eyes are extremely delicate, so you could hit or scratch the eyes using your fingers or other sharp objects. This can cause your opponent to be blind for a time and permit you to get away. Also, the nose can be delicate and is easily damaged. The most effective method to hit the nose is to strike from the bottom, which will cause anyone to tear up and experience shooting pains. You can strike with the palm's bottom or your elbow to hit. Ears are also very delicate and easily struck and not cause damage to the ears.

The neck is the place where major veins and arteries are in addition to serving as breathing passageway. The neck is a target that can temporarily cause your attacker to be unconscious. Stopping oxygen and circulation to this area can leave any person unconscious for a short period of time.

The knee is weakened at any angle. You could directly strike it with your lower body that is, in the case of the majority of women, is usually more powerful than the upper. You can strike your opponent's knee from either side or behind to cause him to lose balance. The knee's front is great to strike as well, but it won't cause any injury as badly.

The groin is known as the most vulnerable area and a severe strike to it can leave anyone in a state of unconsciousness. It is

possible to punch or kick at the groin, then
sprint away in search of safe.

Chapter 12: Comfort Of Home Safety

Every person, regardless of age or gender is likely to claim that their safest spot is at home. Home is the place we associate with words such as security, comfort as well as many others. That's exactly what it ought to be. But, we recognize that this isn't always the situation. This is where the home security measures come into play. There could be situations where an intruder or any other person attempts to break into your home in a violent manner and attempt to cause harm. By taking the appropriate steps to protecting your home can make it easier to avoid these situations generally. Making sure your family and home are secure should be your top first priority. This is especially true especially for women who live on their own as they are more likely to be the target of the kind of privacy invasions that can occur. By taking a few simple steps every day and protecting your home in a more secure manner will go a long ways in making your home secure and will put you secure and at peace.

Essential home security measures

The following are a few essential steps to make sure the safety of your house secure home:

Securely lock your doors no matter if you're in your home or going out. If you're not going to be home, be sure that all windows and doors securely secured, especially if windows are not barricaded. Many people neglect their back doors, as well as those in the garage. These doors provide easy for burglars trying to break into your home.

• Keep the lights in the best possible condition. Burglars tend to avoid places that are well lit. Keep the lights off when you are out in the city, and usually signal that your house is empty to them.

Be sure to never leave keys outside. Anyone trying to enter the house will first search for keys under the doormat.

* Signs such as "Beware of Dogs" actually aid in keeping off unwelcome visitors. The presence of a real dog is more effective than using fake signs.

* Inform a trusted neighbour know when you'll be away and provide their contact information to inform you in the event that they notice something unusual.

Make sure you invest in a top door lock that is of high-quality. Also, consider investing in a quality alarm system from a reputable company. It will activate an alarm when an intruder attempts to gain entry into your home. It is important to ensure that your family members know how to set off the alarm. Choose a security provider that has the highest response times.

Note: Don't leave an entry on your door so that people can know when you're out because this could be a good sign to burglars. They also have a knack of watching the home, and if they are hearing the phone ring continuously but not being heard, they could conclude that nobody is at in the house. This is why it is important to lower the volume of your caller while away.

Make sure your mailbox is locked so that nobody else is able to access any mail which may contain personal information.

The addition of motion sensor lighting on your outdoor lawn or area will help in the evening.

* Be aware of sales managers. Avoid them as much as you can. Don't give your door to anyone you don't know. Don't divulge your personal details to anyone who claims to be any or your providers. Contact the company and verify to see if they have provided someone.

Chapter 13: Street Weapons For Self Defense

The most common street weapons are weapons that you can hide easily, allowing users to carry them easily in the event of need. Staffs and swords are excellent weapons, but you'll not be able to conceal them inside your clothing. Carrying large weapons around can not only create terror in the community, but can also draw an eye of the police officers and other law enforcement officials.

There are a variety of street weapons to choose from and they are available on the internet or at your local outdoor retailer. These are the most well-known weapons can be easily hidden inside your bags and wear everyday:

Pocket folding knife. This knife is not just ideal for stabbing and slashing in self-defense situations and is ideal as a multi-purpose tool. It's small enough to be carried in a pocket. The drawback of it is it's prohibited for carrying in certain areas.

A pocket butterfly knife. This knife was developed from Southeast Asia. It functions similarly to the pocketknife but it can be closed and opened with ease. This particular method of exposing and hiding the blade is used to prevent accidental cutting the hand or fingers. Like the pocketknife it is prohibited to carry in certain places.

The Credit Card Knife. It is a tiny but extremely effective knife that can serve as a self-defense weapon as well as it is a multi-purpose tool. Its unique design makes it simple to hide. You can transform it into a flat piece card that is as large as a credit-card and the same thickness as two credit card when stacked together. You can put it in your wallet so that law enforcement officers will not be able to determine that you have concealed the weapon.

Kubotan Keychain. The unique tool is legally legal in all regions. The self-defense keychain is less than six inches long and half one inch in diameter. It has an attached keyring that can be used for additional concealment and comfort for the user. Due to the key ring, the kubotan is seen as a regular keychain to most people who is looking at it. On the other side of the kubotan has an abrasive point that is which is designed to put pressure on the most sensitive areas of an adversary's body. It is also possible to use the weapon with precision with key chains hanging. In this situation, use the keys attached to the direction of an adversary to disorient him.

These are just a few examples of self-defense weapons can be used on the streets. Remember that they are all in small sizes, they're efficient in close-quarter combat.

Chapter 14: Simplicity

Anything you do to ensure the safety, security and property of your family and family members is valuable. Even if it is feasible with one simple object or reckless method, it is a sign that you've done the thing required to defend yourself. It is not necessary to appear as a hero of legend and engage in a fight with the criminals blood for blood or tooth against tooth, or carry a gun or knife in all at all times. Simple means "ending the threat in the best method you can" by using the most simple and most efficient method you can think of.

How? You could do this by avoiding fighting with a person in traffic, as well as not making a major issue of a conversation with someone who is trying to get ahead of the line despite your courteous warnings. Or if you suspect you are attacked or your vehicle, you should remain in the vehicle or calling police leaving the scene, or if you're in your home, make sure you keep your doors locked and remaining in the house. You can make use of a chair to act as an obstacle for keeping the attacker's weapon or knife from your reach or, if you spot someone suspiciously approaching you, you should immediately leave the area.

You can see that the key to success is having a simple designed plan by selecting the most effective method for the various stages of attitude as well as skills and plan. It all depends on your understanding, wisdom, and certainly your previous discussions and studies on this subject i.e. your spiritual, emotional, and psychological training. By learning simple methods that have been tested and used by people who have been through real-life events and will expand your horizons.

Weapons Around Us

Our country is a place in which carrying firearms and sharp objects is prohibited by the law. It is quite likely that we won't be able to locate the right weapon or object to protect ourselves. (Even the case and do, it might get us in trouble with police). If we do examine our surroundings with care our surroundings are packed with potential weapons. A mop, hanger stone, chair tree branch, table salt, sand etc. Anything that is available could be utilized to defend yourself in the event in need. In the section "Barriers and obstacles" it is possible to protect ourselves and maintain our distance from the attack, or to attack using an enormous object and then throw back what is directed at us.

The ability to defend yourself does not just depend on the situation within your immediate vicinity during the time of attack and the extent to which you can use your mind and wit, but also by understanding defensive strategies, watching actual videos, and learning from the experience. The sound of screaming and shouting can draw attention to help, while also provoking the criminals (at at least for a short time) and eventually leading to their retreat. This allows you to choose as well as the chance to flee and escape.

If You're in Your Car

What are you to do in the event of the possibility of robbery attempts on your valuables in or around your vehicle? Absolutely, the most effective defensive device and method to defend against attack on or around your vehicle is your vehicle. It can be used as a protection. If you are able to increase your awareness and recognize the threat approaching and get to your vehicle and secure those doors (new generation cars come with an all-door lock button)in time, you'll be able to secure your family and yourself from criminals.

If you're strapped in within your vehicle, take off your seatbelt immediately. If you're able to get your car and then drive toward them, you could get out of the danger zone and run over attackrs, thus putting an end to an imminent threat.

The Covering and Concealing of the Crime

This chapter will show the reader how to deflect an attack when you are within the attack's range as an addition to the strategies described in section Barricades and Impediments.

If you're caught in the center of a war and are unable to flee, be lying on the ground immediately or retreat behind a wall in order to shield yourself. Most people freeze in the situation and become scared, not knowing what they should do, which can make you a prime target for shooting.

Women, in particular, should carry their bags across the aisle and with their backs facing the road to avoid purse-snatching. This will stop drag due to the opposition to purse-snatching.

to enter or not to Step In

It's a little difficult understanding what we should do as an observer in the midst of disputes between parties[51[51. What should we do if we witness someone being targeted? Should we step into their shoes, breaking the bystander effect, and then step into the scene? Should we just declare "who really cares" and go forward? Are we trying to stop the fight? There are not only human dimensions involved, but there are also logical dimensions. If we are aware of the person who is being attacked and we have something we can do we will surely intervene and stop the fight, or at least safeguard the victim. But what happens when we you don't know who is fighting or their connection to each the other?

Be extra careful when you don't know what the relationship between the parties is to one another. This could be a kind of circumstance that you shouldn't engage in. If you don't, you may be found guilty. It could be a domestic dispute, or father-son conversation. In these instances, knowing when and when to intervene is crucial not only for the protection of the parties who are involved but also for the safety of witnesses. A fight that escalates to the danger of one person should be avoided at all costs. If you witness a situation like this, you should call the police since they're infringing on the peace of the public. However, if you notice an imminent danger, employ any of the options (if you are unsure of the best technique) that are listed here to get into the situation!

In previous articles the drawbacks of being a witness (nowadays there is a trend to capture videos of events using smartphones). The best course of option is to move away from the area of danger or take cover to ensure self-defense.

Firearm Security

The most important thing to remember for enemies or friends is to recognize that a firearm is "a dangerous tool" and to never play jokes with guns and to abide by the rules of safety for firearms[5252. There have been stories on the news about numerous deaths due to such jokes or in ignorance of the gun lock. In addition, there are tragedies at weddings that result from accidental shooting...

The gun must be secured, using the trigger finger near the trigger instead of pressing the trigger. Guns must be kept from children's reach and shouldn't be used for cleaning when they are present. Anyone who has a job that requires the recourse to guns, for example the police or soldier, or hunting or for sports, must be wary of pointing the gun at someone even if they are laughing.

In the event of a threat or emergency in the event of threats, a warning shot[53is not allowed to be fired at the sky. Warning shots should be fired on the ground or in another suitable location. Don't forget the amount of victims who have died by gunshots that have been fired randomly is not less than a certain amount!

If you shoot or point your gun at an person who is attacking you to defend yourself, make sure that there is no innocent person who is in the area becomes a subject to attack. Gunshots from random fire can strike any other person around, but not the attacker. Such inattention could make you a criminal under the law. It is certain that it will take innocent lives!

Fundamental First Aid Skill

We believe that after eliminating a risk and securing the area that we and our family members (sometimes those who were the perpetrators) are able to survive the incident suffering injuries. We've put up an effective fight, we have stopped the attacker from attacking us or the attacker has succeeded in attacking us or stealing our belongings and then fled.

Most important we can do for the rest of the victims (and certainly for us) is to be at a steady pace and provide basic first aid, without ever giving up (of of course we will need to learn the necessary abilities).

We must call or inform others to dial the emergency number which is 112 for the country we live in. It is suggested to pronounce it as "call 1-1-2 One 2!" There are a lot of people who complain about not receiving an ambulance after dialing 100102 and were told to dial "one one hundred twelve" is not just a few). For the US it is 911 (nine one).

We could have been wounded, pierced, or cut. We're bleeding. The first step is to apply pressure to the area of bleeding with our hands. It is crucial that we keep the first-aid tools in reach [54Then, we should apply pressure to the bleeding. If there is no first aid equipment is readily available, we must cover the wound with a piece cloth, if that is possible. If that is not feasible it is recommended to continue applying pressure. It is important to try to keep our breathing steady and then unlock the door to let emergency services in. We should then wait just in front of the door to ensure that emergency personnel can locate us in case we faint or become unconscious.

It is simpler to stop bleeding from venous sources. But blood flows out of the arteries, making it challenging for a patient to cease bleeding. A patient may end up dying if a tourniquet not used within one or two minutes. A knife cuts arteries, or a blow at the heart can cause death.

Be aware that we must be well-equipped with the basics of first aid not just for emergencies at the outside but also for a variety of situations at work, at home and in the house as well as for our family members. Join first aid classes in your area. Health authorities in your area and some security and medical companies offer such training for free.

IN SUMMARY: Simplicity

Utilize your wisdom/wit[55Apply your knowledge and wisdom[55

Make use of the tools we have around us [56Use the tools around us[56

Defensive tools (force multipliers)

Using your tools effectively

Keep tool on you (firearm, pepper spray, knife, bat etc.)

First aid skills to apply

Chapter 15: The Fight

Despite all your efforts to stop an incident however, you are in a situation where you have to fight for safety. Knowing how to strike will help you safely home.

There are numerous ways strikes can be integrated into self-defense, either in a preemptive or a proactive. Strikes are most effective when using all of your body in order to target the most vulnerable parts of your opponent. It is important to integrate all as our legs, hips and core as we can into every strike. We accomplish this by turning our shoulders and hips throughout each movement. When we combine the amplified gross motor ability of adrenaline and the correct technique, it results in extremely powerful striking.

Some of the most danger-prone targets likely to be:

*chin/jaw

*groin

*throat

*ears

*face(area beneath the eye brows)

Certain body parts are prone to being targets for sensitivity, like the liver or the solar plexus. However we will focus on the areas which are the easiest targets to strike under tension.

Many strikes are removed from this book, including the punch. The use of punches as a method for self-defense can be a valuable benefit. However, it could also be a danger. An injury that is common can result from poor punching technique, referred to as boxer's fracture. A boxer's fracture occurs when the 5th or 4th metacarpal bones of the hand break typically from striking an object or a person. It's for this reason that I've decided not to protect this strike.

How do I train at home?

If you intend to exercise at home with your family or friends, make certain to be cautious. You must ensure that everyone is sufficiently warmed up and have were cleared by their physician for any physical activity.

Some notes:

A proper warm-up should cause your joints to feel loose and you should feel an occasional sweat.

Make sure you exhale while you strike so that your body is able to process oxygen. It's okay if the exhale takes either a grunt, or growl. In fact, it'e better if if does.

If feasible, I suggest an appropriate pad designed to be held in order to strike. Professional quality pads can be purchased online through Amazon. Facebook Marketplace can provide access to previously used pads for cheaper prices. You can also use household products instead of pads. Whatever you choose to use, be sure it's solid enough to provide them with resistance and not harm the pad holder when it comes into contact.

Intensity is crucial in this case however, it's not at all as much as frequency. If you train only one time and at 100%, it doesn't work as well as doing repeatedly over several weeks or even months, at 50% intensity.

1.When you are first learning about the strike, be sure you practice it slowly for at least a duration of a. When you're more confident in your technique, you will be able to increase the level of intensity. There are plenty of ways to learn this, but we'll concentrate on making it easy.

A. Warm-up period of about one minute for each strike. This gives the pad holder as well as the striker the chance to be adjusted.

B. Let's increase the speed. From 100 percent, your drilling power is about 70 percent. If you are drilling, aim 30 seconds of hitting, then 30 seconds of relaxation.

After that you may switch to your partner or continue with the drill.

C. After you have completed 2-3 sessions of this, you should stop for a moment. The break can last up to a minute or for as long as it is necessary to replenish your heart rate and breath. It is important to stay hydrated.

D. This time, you're working at full force and putting everything into it. Be sure to exhale each time you hit. The goal is 20 seconds of hard work and then 10 seconds of rest to complete 3-4 rounds.

2. After working on all the strike-related skills It's time to focus on self-defense.

*Remind the protector to make the defense, and then getting away. We must develop the habit of getting safely quickly.

* Strike as hard as you can (making sure you don't strike the person you are with). If the attacker falls or is awed by the strikes, get up and run. A single strike is rarely enough to stop an attack, however.

Attack the targets of the attacker (chin jaw, throat) until it's safe to leave.

If you fail to play your defense during drilling, don't give up. It is essential to develop the mindset of overcoming errors. It's not about being perfect but rather getting involved.

A. Do each self-defense exercise for about 5-8 minutes per. Change roles each attack and your other partner, as necessary.

B. After you've covered every aspect of the self-defense strategies, make it more interesting by allowing the attacker to make use of any of the techniques you have studied. The key is that the defense must begin each attack by closing their eyes. When they feel the threat, they are able to open their eyes and begin the defense. Keep your eyes shut. We're not training to become Ninjas.

Eyes closed can make this an extremely stressful experience for the protector.

Security note: Attackers are aware that your opponents have their eyes shut. If you are too aggressive and forcefully hitting your hands on their throat or pressing them with an accordion could likely cause injuries.

"The body can't move in a direction where the mind hasn't been first. "Brian Stuart Germain. Brian Stuart Germain

The phrase works both ways. Your mind is able to plan the entire day long, but until you are feeling the strain of your training, the chance is very low that you'll respond similarly under stress.

Chapter 16: Common Self-Defense Mistakes to Avoid

Don't attack the groin correctly The groin of the attacker is usually thought of as a quick and effective method of gaining an advantage, this does not mean all you have to do is throw a punch or kick, and then let the nature take care of the rest. There's actually an art to striking the groin area than you would think. It is, first and foremost you must meet up close to the person you are aiming at when going to the groin area, because the greater distance between you and your attacker, the higher the likelihood that you'll either hit them or be able to counter the strike. Additionally, once you've gone for the groin one time the attacker is likely to be more cautious within that region, meaning it is likely that you won't be able to take another shot that is clear unless you're fortunate. Be sure to get close enough to make the most of your strike.

It is also important not to fall into the trap of tackling the groin area head-on in the event that you are able to steer clear of it. This is because once you strike, the body's natural reflex to spinal pressure will begin to kick in. This is a reflex that causes the body in order to protect itself , without conscious thought in this situation it causes the hands to lower to shield the area that is inflicted and the upper body will begin to bend. The knees will begin to collapse and the chin will be splayed out.

Although this can make ending the fight much simpler If you're directly facing your adversary, this gives them the perfect chance to headbutt you from their new place. Be sure to put your feet slightly away to ensure you aren't impacted when performing what you must do. When you strike it, you'll need to move your body at approximately 30 to 45 degrees so that you are outside the zone of impact.

To make sure an erect groin attack effective it is crucial to draw your attacker into the illusion of security before. Take a few minutes to attack other areas before you distract the attacker towards the potential of a strike . This will make sure that when you head to the targeted area you will strike.

In general, you should to begin with strikes to the head or neck to move the attacker forward so that you can align a good shot with less difficulty. Head blows also could confuse or stun your attacker and make the task you have to do more simple. After you have gotten several blows to the head, your adversary's attention tends to be on protecting the head which means that it is less likely that they'll be able to move and deflect the attack.

In the end, it's crucial to always be prepared with a backup plan to follow-up if the strike to the groin is expected and causes your attacker to stop. Rememberthat the attacker is likely to be riding high on adrenaline, so even firmly contacting to your shin isn't likely to keep them from escaping for long. Moreover, they're likely to be with more determination to commit violence as they did prior to. It is essential to be aware of whether you intend to use your advantage or attempt to make a run to avoid it prior to making your move, so you get as much time to execute your plan as quickly as you can. Rememberthat you've just gained control of the situation you have landed a blow like this so be ready to leverage it to the fullest extent.

In the dark about the right time to end a fight It is vital to remember that any fight that involves an unknown opponent is likely to result in serious injury or death, and therefore fight according to that, it's equally crucial to remember that no fight have to come to either of those outcomes. The truth is that when a fight has clearly ended your way there are a variety of ways to stop the situation from spiralling until everyone would be happy in the event that it didn't happen.

The first thing to do is when you can use a lot of force against your opponent in a short time, it's likely that they'll reconsider the initial attitude of a hostile one. Sometimes, simply showing the other person that you're not someone to be taken lightly, or that you will be easily intimidated can make them make them reconsider their position, provided you offer them a means to leave the situation with ease. In this regard, it's ideal to apply pressure consistently and continuously for a long time to establish your power and then give the other party with an opportunity to leave the situation in a peaceful manner. If you give them with this chance and they continue to attempt to engage against you, you may continue the fight to its logical conclusion being confident that you provided them with the chance to be safe from injury.

Making the wrong move: Although you must always try to stay clear of a fight whenever feasible, there will be a moment when it's obvious that a fighting will occur regardless of what you do. In this situation it is crucial to be proactive and take the first step in order to not end up as the one who winds getting injured, or even worse. Over 50 percent of the time, a battle is decided by the one who makes the first punch. If a fight must be fought, you must be this person as often as you can.

It is also crucial that if you're fighting, you are completely committed to the conflict. When the adrenaline begins to flow and you are unable to predict what the other side might take action, so any hesitation could result in serious negative effects. Don't allow the other party to decide the outcome, and when it's time for rubber to be driven take your time and remember your lesson and demonstrate to them that the choice they made to escalate the situation to the level of violence isn't something that they can repeatedly repeat.

Beware of looking for any additional attackers: If yourself being attacked suddenly without any apparent reason, it's easy to focus your attention on the cause of the attack and ignore everything other. That is one mistake that could probably cost you a lot of money because if the attack is planned, there are likely to be other attackers on the horizon to assist the attacker in case things turn sour for them. Therefore, when you begin a fight, it is crucial to take the time to look around and ensure you are aware of what you can be expecting.

This will enable you to be ready in the event that additional adversaries be discovered, but it will also give you an understanding of any dangers to be aware of or items you can make use of for your benefit. Additionally, you could discover that the opportunity to assistance or stopping the battle before it escalates overly is close to hand. Whatever happens, being aware of your surroundings will prevent you from being caught off guard when the fight gets heated and you're unable to ignore your attackers or the ones you are fighting.

Don't look for fights, even when you think you've had enough experience to be able to manage yourself in all circumstances, it's likely to be a mistake to enter into fighting without having exhausted the other options first. Engaging in a fight you don't really need to is like gambling, and you don't are sure of what's going to occur. Just one lucky strike to cause serious injuries or even death. Being on the other side of that punch will create a lot of stress following the fight. You can avoid a lot of trouble and try to stop the fight before it escalates into violence each time, no matter what.

Don't aim for the stomach. If you're in the middle of a battle it can be difficult to concentrate and select those targets that make the most sense in the circumstance. In any case it is crucial to do the best you can to not waste time kicking your stomach, as 90% of the time it's going to make little difference in securing your adversary while at simultaneously wasting energy and allowing yourself to be vulnerable to a counterattack. The stomach is not a good target generally speaking to be a legitimate goal, instead, focus on your body's weak points instead.

Chapter 17: Selecting The Style Of Study

Synopsis

If you're looking to study the art of fighting there's plenty to learn about the various styles. Naturally, there's the issue of finding the best martial art, an issue that a lot of people ask. With so many different styles of martial art to pick from. It can be a challenge to pick one to study.

The Choice

No matter what you may listen to or what other people might have to say it's difficult to pinpoint one particular style of martial arts as being the most fundamentally superior. There are a lot of elements that play into making a claim that a certain style is the best is a stretch. Although one style may outdo another in a match or fight, it doesn't suggest that the winning method is the most effective.

Before you rush to learn martial arts there are many aspects to consider first.

Around the globe There are a variety of dojos and martial arts classes which emphasize self-defense significantly more than others. Schools that concentrate on forms, kata or sparring in a light manner are not likely to train you in the techniques you'll need to know to stay safe in the street. If you're seeking street self-defense, you'll need a technique that is hard-working and never stop.

Although martial arts can improve your fitness however, that's not the main goal behind the majority of forms of martial art. Some styles, such as Tae Bo, are based exclusively on martial arts, and do not include any physical fitness instruction. If you're seeking fitness as your primary objective it is recommended to consider something other then martial arts.

The ability to fight will differ among the various martial art styles. Self-defense schools often focus on combat techniques, teaching you all you require to be a successful fighter. A lot of martial arts are slow in the theory department and teach you kata as well as movements and forms. Self-defense schools, however can teach you how to do the various kinds of damage in the shortest period of time.

Martial arts that are based on competition are about winning awards and demonstrating to the world your unique style of martial arts. The competition you've picked will significantly impact your martial arts style. It is important to decide whether you'll be fighting or demonstrating display kata heavy or light contact, or focusing on grappling or striking.

Before you choose an art of martial arts it is important to research the dojos and schools in your region and check out what they can offer you. The most reputable schools will allow you to participate in a handful of classes free or offer discounts for the first few months. They'll help you with any questions you may have and will aid you in helping you to learn as much as you want to.

The Wrapping Up

Be conscious of what's happening in the
vicinity - when walking along the street Do
you know that you're being observed?
When you're out walking or running, in a
quiet area and wearing earphones, this are
likely to reduce your alertness.

While walking, keep an eye on the traffic
coming towards you. Make sure your
hands are from your pockets, so that they
are ready to use if you're pulled. Move
with confidence; appear as if you know the
direction you're taking and what you're
headed, even when you don't. Keep your
eyes up and your head down.

Have you seen a car pass by your home a
number of times? Or perhaps someone
sitting in front of your school or
workplace. Adults do not have to be asking
kids for help. It's safer to be in a group.
Avoid walking through dark areas or
alleyways for a quick escape. Always
inform others of where you are , and at
the time at which you plan to be there. Be

sure to trust your guts, if you spot something strange occurring, you should avoid it and inform someone about it.

If you are walking or running in a group, don't use headphones. Do not answer inquiries from strangers via phone by stating that you're on your own. Engage individuals in a manner that makes them are aware that you've seen them (a potential crook wouldn't like to be identified, making them more likely to seek. assistance, yourself.

It is a good idea to shout out loud so that someone can be at your door if for there's nothing else to do; at the very least, you're drawing attention to them. Don't ride along. Be cautious when using ATMs at evening. If you carry a bag with a strap , make sure you set it so that you can let the bag go when it's stolen and you get injured in the event that you're being dragged along by it.

If a stranger comes up to you and asks for directions, keep an appropriate distance from them. If you're taking someone to their house, ensure they're inside safely before you leave. If you're a solo driver and notice an accident or stranded driver make a report on your mobile phone or the nearest phone.

Make sure you do your exercises at home with close friends or family members or attend classes, look for more information and don't ignore the psychological or verbal aspects. Create the confidence you're confident in yourself and that you're prepared for self-defense. Take control of your destiny instead of leaving it in the hands of an envious killer.

Chapter 18: Stand-Up Fighting Skills

In a fight in a fight, it is important to "always be moving to be alert and avoid sitting still, and changing your posture; [36] be sure to watch always your rear". Fixed targets are susceptible to attack. Particularly, being active and not allowing yourself to stand still are more crucial in assaults with guns.

Do you remember those documentaries about animals that you might have seen at one point. Animals begin by aiming at the game's throat, and then choke it. They stop them from playing, and make it unstable by constant and circular motions.

Humans are also guilty of this. If you stop breathing the moment you stop breathing, you're finished. If you are unable to move and do not move, then you're an inactive duck. This is also true for the attacker. Whatever strength the attacker is, any hit at his eyes using your fingers or nails and any attempt to poke his face, or even

116

strike to the ear or throat of his opponent can deter him. Moving into your opponent's blind spot i.e. his back when fighting will help you to. Even when you're to the floor, you can kick and stomping to hit your tibia, testicles, and if you have been able to lean back enough that his face is highly efficient.

Ground Fighting Skills

It is generally believed that a stand-up battle continues in this manner for a time but it then transforms into a ground battle (if it continues) whether with weapons or hand-to hand combat. In cases of rape it's already the goal of the attacker to put the victim down. It is of utmost importance to learn "Stand-Up and Ground fighting Skills" for stand-up and ground combats that don't require kicks or punches (The most popular martial art that trains defense techniques for ground combat can be described as Ju-Jitsu). In reality an attack while lying standing on the floor or leaning against the wall can be more effective against an attacker. Imagine an attacker crashing his face against flooring or against the wall, while certain parts that are part of you shielded by the floor or the wall...

If an attacker attempts to hit you with a kick or with an object after you are in the floor, it is best to avoid or block him with our feet and then get up from the ground as quickly as we can to avoid these attacks and, consequently, ensure our vital organs are protected[3737. In the event that you are forced to fight with your attacker upon the floor, be sure you strike his face and eyes to avoid the most basic and frightening attacks.

In actuality ground defense is actually an altered pivot of stand-up defense strategies. Also the stand-up defense methods are vertical (on the Y Axis) while ground defense methods are horizontal (on the X Axis) in a more restricted method. Imagine apply these techniques on the ground, rather than being leaning vertically on the walls. (Figure 8)

It is also important to note that "ground and lying upon the floor" is crucial in the case of abduction and kidnapping. Your body mass causes you to remain in place because you are unable to walk with your legs (just as wheels) and , consequently, lowers the chance of being kidnapped. If you are able to kick with force and resist, the risk decreases further. "The importance of having feet in the air" will increase since it not only become possible to block and repel the attacker , but also grab the body or head of the attacker with legs and then push him away using your feet, a bigger hand than your hands as in Jui-Jitsu and Ninjutsu.

Figure 8. Foot fighting, and its importance

Skills for Falling

Let's suppose that you've been pushed, tripped , or dropped to the ground during the start of or during a battle. You tumble down...Or let's say it's not an attack, but you fall on the floor that is wet or on snow, or on ice...Yes the floor is mostly concrete, and the road is asphalt, therefore how do you safely fall without being injured?

There are a variety of techniques to help you fall that doesn't result in damaging your head to the ground or falling on your joints that don't cause injury to them. They also enable you to get up quicker than you did when you fell. These techniques are dependent on the speed of your fall and include forward, lateral and backward methods, and so on. You can fall safely without being injured and quickly return to upright posture even in a firm surface, however it requires constant effort in the fitness center. Learning requires exercising. These techniques, particularly are part of the realm of martial arts, such as Judo, Ninjutsu and Ju-Jitsu. This book is not a comprehensive guide to the in-depth explanations for these techniques.

5D's and 1 in Self-Defense

What can you do to get away from someone who is holding a sharp or penetrating object, such as the screwdriver, knife gun or hammer? If you believe that you aren't competent or in any way able to escape , you also don't intend to be killed in the moment, instead you plan to fight. Are you going to attack him to grab his head or wrap your body around him?

Numerous real-life incidents show that the victim lashes out the attacker, then clenches his hands and fights the attacker. The victim typically clenches his the attacker's head, body and throat, and then wrestles with his body, while the danger of a knives is evident and the attacker's swift hand is always ready to cut the victim to pieces. This same risk is apparent when carrying any type of sharp objects or firearms at close range. (Figure 9)

Figure 9. 5D's plus 1 rule in self-defense

One of the first ways to protect yourself from an attack who holds or carrying a knife, gun or comparable weapon would be to limit and, if necessary, eliminate the harm caused by weapon. This is known as "5D's one rule of self-defense[38[38]]". The 5D's in this mnemonic are referring to 5 actions which begin orthographically with the letter "D."

These are the 5 steps that follow:

Deflect

Dominance

Distract

Disarm

Disable

While Plus 1 refers to the "Distance" which must be considered at every step, and should always be maintained separated from the attacker. FiveD's Plus 1 Rule is paramount importance when it comes to self-defense, and it is a simple tool to remember during training. We'll now look at the method step-by step.

1. Deflect

Check the distance first before moving the gun barrel or knife away from your vital organs. The knife should be far away from your body or throat and the gun shouldn't shoot at you anymore.

2. Dominance

Check that the knife or gun isn't pursuing a path that could again lead towards your vital organs and then engulf the knife. The attacker will not be in a position to point the weapon or the gun at you.

3. Distract

Assuming we've successfully taken on the attacker's weapon although the barrel isn't able to shoot towards you at this point but the attacker holds the knife or gun with a firm grip. He is trying to take advantage of this weapon to kill you off. Thus, you have to deflect the attacker from the hand by making an impact that could cause the attacker a sudden discomfort or even an injury. These tiny impacts are called "shocking". If you can distract the person attacking you away from the weapon, and from engaging in a battle by holding a gun and it becomes simpler for you to grab the weapon.

4. Disarm

Remove the attacker from his knife or gun to ensure that he is not able to use the weapon against you. Since he's not armed the attacker is able to cause minimal harm.

5. Disable

Disabling means removing the attacker's capabilities to the maximum extent possible and completely preventing any imminent threat. It could mean mutilating, blocking or even killing the attacker, based on the type of the attack and the incident.

We have already explained that Distance, as Plus 1, implies that you have to control the distance before everything else to take place. The ability to maintain distance in check is essential that helps safeguard our vital organs.

Force Multipliers/Strengtheners

Before you apply the skills and techniques employed during this "Physical fitness and skill" phase, consider the use of any weapons or tools, as well as force multipliers. Also that the use of instruments and tools referred to in the field of "defensive tools" should be the primary strategy to protect yourself from attacks as per the saying "a bad worker is responsible for its tools". For instance, it is important that you carry pepper spray a readily accessible manner - at least within your reach or in the form of either a knife, bat, or gun[39] or if none of them are available, "to use the things around" and then to come up with a way to utilize them in the event of a threat (like drivers who have the jimmies under their seats). If none of the above is accessible, then you are strongly encouraged to shout and shout in many instances. A loud voice can alert and shock the person who is attacking. It is therefore beneficial for you to have a whistle on your keychain, and to carry it around in times of emergency.

"To utilize whatever that we own, even if they're simple objects" such as chairs, makes it possible to defend against the knife that attackers use. A dress hanger could be used as bats. Throwing a spall or container like a tin can is ideal. If we're inside an automobile that is locked, locking it could be beneficial for offensive and defensive purposes. In short, we have to know "how to use effectively our tools and instruments". Again, it's essential to "keep the gun or tool of the attacker (knife or bat, firearm, etc.).) in check and out of our reach" or at a minimum, be aware of this.

It is certainly important to have the right tools for defense. However, what's most vital to consider is "carrying these tools in all at all times". It doesn't matter if you put these instruments in the pocket of your bag, hidden in a drawer, inside a glove box in your vehicle or in the back of the car "away of your own body". These tools are "force multiplyers" only when they are combined with physical capabilities and strength, so as to increase the force needed to defend against an attacker. When fighting, first you must be in a good state of mind "to know your strength and resistance". If you are carrying a gun, you should be the one "to take the first shot or the first to attack" and again to struggle with the attacker using chemical irritants, which may be commercially-available sprays salt or detergent, and pepper spray, Otherwise, you might need to refer to your defense skills.

Multiple Attackers/Attacks

It is important to consider the guardians of attackers/response from standing forces Multiple attacks i.e. battery, robbery and kidnapping of multiple people from at the beginning of an attack. However, it can be more difficult to deal with "multiple attack participants". There is always the possibility that "third actors, attackers, or third parties are involved" in the attack.

For instance an armed robber might have a supporter and a friend who are watching for his. It is important to "check the surroundings for potential dangers". Our endurance and strength should be far more than is needed to fight an individual adversary. Our determination and tenacity should be are, too.

In these situations it is important to be aware of the other attackers when fighting with the other, "using the primary attacker himself as the shield" to avoid attackers as well as to take on attackers (in this scenario one attacker will be in the back of another). There are a variety of methods to use, such as hitting one opponent while throwing things towards the other, or protecting ourselves by using a captured weapon could be employed. Keep in mind that it's not feasible for more than 10 people to attack the identical person simultaneously in the course of a battle. There's not enough room to do this. It is important not to fall down, but to get rid from them, and to show determination and demonstrate resistance. You should also consider the value to your physical capabilities or defense tools.

But, be aware that "unarmed resistance to multiple robbers or attackers (without forces multipliers) is ineffective[42[42". If you're unarmed each strike you make at attackers should disarm or disarm the attacker, in order to be able to take on the next attacker since your strength will weaken and will eventually cease.

until the Threat actually stops

If you think you've escaped the danger and stopped the attacker, be cautious and exercise security and make sure the threat has been gone away. If it has, aim your weapon at the attacker and tell that he must stop and remain still and keep your distance towards the threat. You must remain in this position until the police or backup forces arrive. One scenario that could alter this is if the team members of the attacker are still around and alive, or should they be waiting to strike yet again.

Another scenario is known as F.I.B.S.A[43Effect, in which the person who is attacked pretends to have been shot and yells "I'm shot!". In this instance it is important to be cautious when approaching the attacker lying on the ground. You should make it clear that any threat to your life has been quelled and that the person who is threatening is actually shot, and the gun is safely out of reach. The most crucial thing to do when you approach your attacker on the ground, you must move the knife or gun away from a distance that can be reached with his hand (if feasible, push the weapon away with your feet).

Pressure Test

A majority of those who are trained in self-defense would like to believe that their self-defense skills can be able to save them from harm if they find themselves in a situation of attack. While martial arts are a great way to build physical strength and defend methods, actual life is quite different. You will never be attacked by an opponent with a predictable pattern or uses a particular technique. This is what happens in gyms. As we train, the attacker attacks us in a regular and unpredictably pattern, and is extremely brutal. But, since we can't be out in the street and provoke others to determine the effectiveness of what we've learned, how do be able to test our skills? How can we improve the endurance of us against these intermittent and unstoppable attacks?

The method is known as"pressure test" or "pressure testing" or the exercise is referred to as"a pressure test.. It is also called "sparring" within martial disciplines like Box or Kick-box, as well as Wing Chun; and as "randori" in Japanese martial arts such as Judo and Aikido. It is an exercise match. Someone or more will target you and apply pressure to your body for the purpose of practicing. This assault could be non-armed or with a knife or bat, depending on the method you are working on. It could also be a freestyle. As a defensive player it is necessary to defend or wrestle using constant smacks and use the strategies you've learned can determine your degree of interiorization of the techniques as well as your endurance in the body. It is also a great aerobic exercise. It's fun, but make sure not to be laughing. Think of it as an actual attack. It is a shift from the theory to the actual practice. Make sure you practice it regularly!

Back Up Plan / Plan B

A backup plan refers to the fact that you previously have already taken "useful precautions to protect yourself". For instance, closing the doors, if there are any in a building or closing an open windows that might permit intrusions into your house, including the door or exit from which you may be protected in the event of an unplanned attack. If your work area requires direct contact with others, (such as a cash desk) installing security barriers or keeping the door to your office closed can protect you from any potential problems.

You must get out of the Danger Zone As Fast as You Can.

No matter if you're alone or with your family members or with family members, you should get out of danger as quickly as you can and avoid returning to the zone of danger for any reason[44[44]. The main objective should be to reach safety promptly [45and safely.

Do not let your weapon go (force multipliers) before the threat is approaching[4646. Keep an eye on the threat (if you've resisted or blocked the attacker) up until police, or a the backup force arrives. Remain vigilant.

Don't chase a fleeing attacker!

Do not chase after an escaping attacker who you might have defeated [47or beaten[47. Particularly, if the issue concerns money or property, let the person go. Your life, your honor and your family are more important.

If, for any reason, it is essential to pursue the suspect you must decide whether or not to pursue. You might encounter an ambush during the next stages of your search. The criminal's accomplices might be waiting in the background to assist.

Protect or Punish?

We've previously mentioned that we could be considered criminals according to legal law in the event that we fail to adhere to the concept of proportionality or equality since it is legal to engage in the act to self-defense[4848. Sometimes, a weak or inexperienced attacker or robber can be stopped by a skilled defensive. The defender is able to slap the attacker. If we want to escape danger and take the attacker away We must understand what is the "difference between security and punishment"[49and not force the victim to refrain from all actions that could render us criminals under the law.

The notion of equality and proportionality could be so vast and bizarre that we have seen or watched on nightly news of a mother throwing her son's slippers or someone throws peaches on her neighbour or even an adult dad throwing bottles of plastic at their son, resultantly getting sent to prison and sent home! Any personal matter regardless of whether charges are dismissed because of the person who was victimized, will under the law, be an official case where the defendant is tried and sentenced.

IN SUMMARY: Margin , and distance

The importance of having a margin/distance threats/keeping and limiting the distance [5050

A defensive posture

Fences that protect

Using barriers

Don't ignore any threat that could be coming your way.

Distractions

Refusing to be kidnapped

Physical fitness

Skills that are not fully developed.

Understanding your strengths

The first step is to shoot on the target

Combating chemical irritating chemicals

What is/isn't deadly force?

There is just a few minutes to react to the attacker

Grappling/Ground Skills

The importance of your feet when you fall or while kidnapping.

Multiple attackers

Third party interactions

In search of additional threats

Chapter 19: Body Language Awareness

Non-verbal and body language are crucial to self-defense. The majority of modern research suggests that up to 55 percent of our communication happens non-verbally. Our posture and manner of conduct tells an awful lot about how others perceive us. Whatever the case, whether we pay attention or not, we are communicating through our posture and body language throughout the day.

Everyday, you're looking around and quickly filing all the other people into a temporary folder that can be reviewed in the future. A Princeton study claims that first impressions can occur in a fraction of one second[66. Hand position or a tilt of the forehead, an expression of frown or smile. There are a myriad of combinations that can be made.

If lions are hunting on grasslands, they're not searching for the most tough prey that they can come across. They are primarily hunting for those who are old, young, or the weak. The hunt for wildebeests in its peak and ready for battle, leads to poor utilization of energy and time. It could also cause injury or death to the Lion. Human predators are very similar to lions.

If predators of humans are looking to find victims, they search at women who appear be unable to communicate with their bodies, like:

*Slumped shoulders

*No eye contact

*Washing away

*Fidgeting hands

* Soft spoken

Cell Phones

Absolutely, the most benign, yet risky danger towards body language comes from the mobile phone. We all have to check emails or Instagram. In the midst of our phones can blind our eyes, leaving us unaware of the world around us. The body is also forced to a posture that is most closely related to predators. Eyes are down as are shoulders, shoulders arched and feet moving in slow steps. We're like shambling zombies running into objects and people.

The constant use of a mobile phone while walking between our locations can cause us to shift our eyes off of the world that surrounds us. We're no longer in a position to see the possible threats that could be threatening us. If you remember in 2016 the year that Pokemon Go first hit the market the streets were packed with people glued to their smartphones. Not able to stop some pedestrians were being hit by cars while they walked through the streets. This was so bad that it was classified as an emerging health risk behaviour by the NCBI[77.

the mask of Confidence

What is a confident appear? Great posture, good smile, eye contact. This isn't rocket science. It's the body language we are trying to convey in public. If you're not confident enough, natural confidence, you can "fake it until it come to mind." If you're meeting people from a different location for example, like the college campus or at a new job It's a new beginning. If the person you meet for the first time seems confident and speaks confidently in the sense that you are concerned you're confident.

For those suffering with Generalized Anxiety Disorder The intervention of an experienced counselor might be necessary. Numerous universities are increasing their counseling and mental health services. If you are suffering from Generalized Anxiety Disorder or a similar disorder, you may call for help from the Substance Abuse and Mental Health Services Administration by calling 1-800-662-HELP.

Steps to Take

1. When you enter an area be sure to keep your head elevated and look around. Take a look around and observe everyone. When you observe their facial expressions, you can determine the difference between someone who's confident and who appears timid, and who appears like someone who is creepy. Threat scans or assessments are an instrument that police use. Law enforcement officers constantly confront situations where there are a lot of unknowns that require quick judgement calls.

Consider it as an actual game. If you keep playing and win, the more. The benefits are many and include:

A. You begin to become familiar with who's around you whenever you are in a new place.

A. The process of scanning the space will force that you keep your eyes straight and keep eye contact with others as you walk into the room. Scanning mimics the posture that shouts "I don't want to be an enemy."

2-Confidence is often a result of the ability. If you've recently relocated from your home and are now living in a different location, it is likely that you don't have the same group of friends or the same social circle. Find something to do you love to do. It could be a hobby project in addition to working or going to school. These can include:

Join clubs. Theatre, music, photography The list is endless. If you enjoy it, do it.

If you're an athletic athlete during high school, but intend to concentrate on college work Don't be afraid to join intramural teams , or the Crossfit gym(If the school you attend doesn't offer one). You are able to control the amount of commitment.

Volunteering for charitable organizations is rewarding due to the positive impact it can have on other people. It also looks great on job applications to mention volunteering experience on your resume.

Chapter 20: Natural Weapons

Engaging in an unprovoked street fight, or even defending yourself against an attack , can happen within a matter of seconds, which means you can use whatever you consider to be the best weapon at the moment. Sometimes it's an old school fight , where you'll only require two hands and strength in your upper body. In other instances, you may require fancy footwork or even incorporating your head. More violent situations could lead to the recourse to weapons. All of these are considered to be natural weapons.

In reality, anything that is able to cause damage in the event that it is for a goal is viewed as weapon. If, for instance, your goal is to hit somebody in the chest, then your fists have become weapons. If you're trying to escape an attacker who is male and decide to kick them in the groin area, you're using your feet as weapons.

A reminder to women trying to defend themselves from the male attacker. The privates should be the primary goal of attack - go at his balls with as strong a punch as feasible. If you're in a fight by a defender, then you should either strike there , and then grab and crush the privates of his. This may sound cruel, but believe me when I say that you'll want to protect yourself by doing this. The dog will release, stop for a split second and you'll be able to escape to safety.

The majority of people are attracted by stereotyped weapons like knives, guns or Tasers. These are all weapons, but they're not necessarily natural. The natural weapon is a reflection of your. Therefore, the next time you witness someone break an open glass bottle and then show it to someone else and then realize that the innocent person being pointed at is actually threatened by an extremely dangerous weapon.

Your weapons of choice can be utilized in different techniques. If you're participant in a battle which turns into close-range combat it is advisable to master the various hold positions that are pain-free. A pain compliance hold occurs the ability to make use of your attacker's body, and the inability to resist the pain they cause. There are a variety of various methods, but the main elements of this technique is moving an appendage opposite direction from where it is supposed to move. The goal is to accomplish this without damaging any bones or joints.

If compliance with pain doesn't result in a successful street fight, many street fights will become ground fights. In other words, both you and your opponent will end up on the ground, fighting each other. In this situation, you could utilize the ground to leverage to hold the advantage. You can also use restraints or holds to keep the attacker from moving or to exhaust them. It's an ideal moment to try to disarm those who are carrying an external weapon like a gun or knives. In a street fight, the goal is not to be a threat to you. Beyond the weapons you're using, willpower and mental strength will assist you in winning in a fight.

Natural weapons are those you feel comfortable with in the event of a crisis that can protect you from harm. Keep this in mind and it could help you save your life in the future.

Chapter 21: How to Let Go of Fear

Synopsis

The process of releasing and conquering your fears isn't an easy challenge and may be impossible for some people. Fear can leave you in a state of paralysis and make you unable to move or react to the circumstance. Many people are scared to do something different and think twice about it. But, to find something that can bring you complete happiness you must learn the art of letting go of the other things.

What To Do?

To conquer your fear you must follow these steps. When you do this you are able to face anything that scares you.

1. Write down the things that scare you. Do not hesitate when you write everything. It is your right to write anything, for instance, fearing to fall, to be

awed by highs, or to fail, or any other thing that scares you. Write everything down and assign rank to them according to the scale of 1 to 5. The number of ranks you assign to them will be based on how they impact your life in general. Choose 1 for things that help you to feel less afraid and 5 for items that can bring great benefits on your life.

2. Write down the items you don't want to try because you're scared to attempt them. This could mean that you hesitate before allowing the help of others , or that you don't want to move to a different state or city. Note them down, and then apply a similar system as that you used for the list of your worries.

3. Start by identifying the fears with the highest scores, and then those items that you avoid. Consider the reasons you are scared of these items and also the reason that you might be hesitant to face some of these issues. Note down your reasons for your fear and opposition. Create a counter-argument for each one. For

instance, if you are scared of dying due to an airplane crash You can counter the question by thinking about the reality the fact that millions of travelers who fly without a single accident.

4. Imagine that you're doing something that is making you feel scared. Make sure you're doing every movement with a positive mindset. Record everything you see about yourself as well as how you feel following the completion of the exercise. Perform this procedure for each anxiety you've got on your list.

5. Start to let go of your fears and take action that won't make a huge impact on your life. If you realize that everything is fine and everything is in order, it will be much easier to be confident enough to confront the things you used be scared of.

Fear can hinder individuals to develop the ability to have a positive mind and increase mental power. In terms of the self-defense of your psyche one must learn how to overcome your fears. an essential thing. When you take the steps mentioned that are listed above, you'll be able to build a stronger mind that is free of negative thoughts that are triggered by fears. So, why should you be scared since fear is all that is in the mind? Remember that a life that is lived in fear is a life that has not been lived.

Chapter 22: Weapons to Make Use Of for Self-Defense

The ability protect yourself from harm is essential for women. There is no need to be afraid of being attacked. Instead, you can be able to move about with confidence knowing that you'll be able to swiftly confront anyone trying to harm you. There are a variety of methods of self-defense that start with fundamental steps, using weapons, and training at higher levels also. The ability to learn any of them is much better than being in the dark when someone is attacking you. Women might be smaller body than the majority of men however that doesn't necessarily mean they are weaker. If they can master the right actions and employ the correct weapons, no one could ever hurt themselves or body part. This chapter will allow you to learn more about the various weapons that are used to protect yourself. They could be deadly and non-lethal weapon. Also, you should look up the regulations in certain states regarding carrying specific weapons. For example, there are some states in which you aren't permitted to carry a firearm in the event that you want to. In these instances, firearms that are nonlethal can be beneficial to use on a regular basis. All weapons are designed to be used for self-defense. They can be used to gain time to escape, while other weapons can be used to attack a predator with the intention of an actual attack.

Nonlethal weapons

If you're not violent in your nature and you don't enjoy carrying knives or guns There are still alternatives for you.

Sprays of pepper are among of the most useful weapons you can carry around. The right spray can cause the victim a significant amount of pain and can temporarily blind them. This gives you plenty of time to handle the person however you wish or simply get them out of the way.

Mace refers to a tear gas kind of spray. It can cause the attacker to choke and cough but isn't as inflamatory as pepper sprays.

• Stun guns offer a second affordable and effective alternative. The power of a stun gun can hurt even the most powerful of men, and will help you when you are in such a situation.

Tactical flashlights are simple to carry around and useful in many ways. The bright light shines towards the eyes of the attacker, and then it temporarily blinds them. This gives you time to react or to run.

Beanbag guns are an alternative to consider. A well-powered device will blow the wind out of anyone. It's very simple to use and extremely efficient.

* Stun batons can be described as sticks that provide a significant amount of force on the person who is attacking. The top of the device, along with the side of the baton are energized. This is the reason

why an attacker isn't able to take it off your hands and not be also stunned. They're a bit bigger than the other gadgets, but they are quite useful.

In terms of home security, we recommend using a strong baseball bat in the vicinity. This may sound like a cliché however, they can be useful in the event that you suddenly hear a noise at night and suspect that there's an intruder inside the home. A hit to the sound with the baseball bat can knock anyone to the ground or even out.

* A Taser could appear like stun gun, however it's not. It has two electrodes that must be in contact with on the face of the victim to allow the current to pass through. It's more efficient than stun guns in stopping the attacker, however it is more difficult to use since it can't penetrate clothes. However, if you train enough you can use it effectively to disarm an attacker regardless of how tall they are.

Lethal Weapons

If the environment you reside in is hazardous or you're worried about your safety, deadly weapons could be the best choice for you. But, they require more attention than the weapons that we have mentioned previously and are only used following properly trained.

Knives are an essential and convenient choice. The majority of people carry a tiny pocket knife or Swiss-army in their purses or on keys. It is also possible to use an extra-large bladed knife however these aren't ideal to carry around or hide. Small knives for tactical use can be carried wherever and utilized to evade the attacker. They are effective in inflicting harm on the attacker if you are able to make them effective.

* Scarves are a surprising yet highly efficient weapon. You can wear one anywhere and nobody would be able to imagine that you could utilize it to your advantage. Make sure you practice using these weapons quickly, and then you can

employ them as garrotes or to strangle your attacker.

* Tactical pen are easily accessible these days. They look similar to pens, however they can be used to defend against attackers , but cutting or punching holes in them.

When using guns when carrying weapons, it is crucial to be careful. As we said earlier ensure that you are allowed carrying the firearm you want to carry in the zone. Should it not be, then you may encounter a problem with the law in that area. It is also important that you pull out your weapon only in situations of defense when your security is in danger and you'll be able prove this before a judge in the event of a situation. Weapons should never be handled with care and needs some training, with some being more so than others. If you're not confident and comfortable with your weapon could easily be taken and utilized against you. It is also possible to harm the innocent people around you If you're not careful.

Chapter 23: What If It All goes wrong

It's not inherently a sign of weakness to take a risk and run. There are plenty of laughs and jokes about letting yourself go, but fighting is not worth the risk of your life. If you're not certain you'll prevail, or if injured and are unable to continue to defend yourself, you'll be required to escape the attacker as fast as you can. Like in all stages of combat, there's a method to safely retreat.

When your adrenaline rush began to kick in, you must have looked for escape options. If you are in a huge crowd, try to make eye contact with the crowd to see if you could find any help to get out of the incident. Street fights are often a spectator sport. This makes it difficult to get out of an argument, but if it's your only option take advantage of it. After you have discovered an escape route, you'll want to try to remain focused and keeping your eyes on top at your adversaries. If they think they are in the position of having just one moment to not be paying attention, they will take advantage of it.

You can catch your opponent off guard. Make use of misdirection or whatever it is they would like to hear to disorient them. It is also useful for carjacking, mugging or thefts. The trick is to disrupt them so that they're not focused on the target. If they break their focus, it will be much easier for you to escape. If they do strike at you when you try to escape, be aware of the most critical areas that could stop a fight with one strike. Be careful not to strike the areas like the diaphragm or temple. These are some places that, if struck, can and could cause permanent damage making it impossible to escape.

In the end, if all of the strategies for evasion do not perform and you're in a fight with a person who clearly has the advantage, it might be the right time to compromise. When animals are in a difficult position, they can choose to playing dead. We do not. However , we can give up. Place both hands on the table like you're blocking a blow and let the impression that you're tapping out. You don't want to engage in a battle. If someone is only looking for blood, the most effective advice is to put the body into a lying position , protecting all vital organs.

While this might seem like an awful way to get out of an argument, it's difficult to confront an opponent who is not fighting against you. If you've provided them with what they want initially and they're still fighting around, there is no reason to attempt to get out. It is obvious that they do not have any intention of letting you quit. It is therefore more crucial to ensure the health of the vital organs of your body, such as your liver, kidneys and head, to ensure that you do not become totally disabled.

Chapter 24: Physical Conflicts What Should You Do When Everything else fails

What happens if you are able to get to the last letter 'C' and the confrontation turns physical? What happens if an assault occurs and you discover yourself as a victim of a predator who is vicious?

There are still actions you can take. You have the power to control your situation. This chapter will provide you with options in case it comes to a battle you will be able to take the best option in your particular situation.

The first thing to note is that this chapter will not be able to discuss physical self-defense techniques. This chapter will focus on the psychological aspects of self-defense here and strategies that have the goal to keep you alive.

If you're interested in learning the physical movements, I'd suggest you to attend an ordinary martial arts class. (I'm in love with Wing Chun because it's so effective in street fighting.) You can also learn a few basic self-defense techniques and train them on a regular routine, repeating them over and over. It will make it much easier to master them in stressful circumstances.

But, this chapter is about teaching you a few simple techniques that you can employ in the event of an attack to ensure that you emerge alive at the end of the tunnel.

Here are a few of my 'hard and fast' 'survival guidelines' in case you encounter a physical confrontation:

#1: Don't Let yourself be taken to a different location The worst thing you could do. Don't drive regardless of what he claims. Do not go with him even if he says that he'll let you go in the event that you agree to it. Do not use your keys to unlock your door to your apartment to him even if he claims that he will not be coming into your home.

9 times out of 10 the second site is the one where the greatest physical harm occurs. This is where the majority of victims are murdered, raped, or even beaten.

Why? Because a second location is silent and unnoticed without any witnesses. You can bet on that.

If you're walking on the street even if you're in an area that is a bit secluded and there aren't many persons, the attacker has no complete control over the area. It's possible that people will still wander around. There might be cameras in an convenience store or bank that can catch the suspect. This can give an advantage in this situation since he's not completely in control of the location.

If you take him to a second place, you've lost the influence. There's nothing that can help you and he has no reason to harm you. In fact there is more motivation to harm you and perhaps cause your death in order to conceal the wrong he's committed.

#2: Once you make the decision to fight back Continue to Fight All the Way and Continue to Do it until Your Attacker has been disabled

This is a fact that most people don't realize:

If you are hit (or wounded) or stabbed, the majority of attackers will continue to come at you for a few minutes after being struck. It is imperative to complete the task.

If you're attacked , and you decide that this is the time to take action take the initiative and fight to the end. Keep fighting until your adversary is down and has no chance of pursuing you. It's not enough to knee an attacker in the groin and hope it puts him to sleep. It could slow him down, it could even cause him to fall to the ground, but it will not stop him from attacking.

Why?

Because the adrenaline in his body is high, and adrenaline provides people with the ability to be super-strong and endurance.

Adrenaline gives an 80-year old grandmother the strength to pull the car off her five year old grandchild. Adrenaline can give a boxer the ability to take over 100 head blows and continue fighting. Adrenaline allows soldiers to keep pushing on their adversaries even after their bodies have been splattered with bullet holes and shrapnel.

While a one knee on the back may be able to stop an intruder on a normal day however, it's not enough to stop him if the body is pumped with adrenaline.

This is especially difficult for women since it goes in opposition to their worldviews. I have observed this in a lot of women I train in martial arts as well as self-defense. They can fight back but they do not go enough.

It's not over. They must fight their inborn beliefs that say, "Be a nice girl" and "Hurting people is not good." It's good for getting along in daily life, but when it comes to the event of an attack the odds are stacked against you. Your life is on the risk, and you're likely be fighting hard to defend yourself.

One tapping on the groin area of an adrenaline-fueled 250-pounder determined to rape you will not stop him. In fact, it might even enrage him. If you choose to fight, be sure to commit 100.

Continue to fight until you are completely defeated and fight with your arms, legs, voice or head, teeth, purse, or anything else until your attacker is stopped and you're given a chance to escape.

#3: Make a distraction If You're Able If someone is looking for your wallet throw it in one direction and then take a different route. If someone is fighting with you and you are not sure what to say, ask them an irrelevant question. This can disrupt their thinking process and cause them to take a step back so that you can escape.

I am friends with a woman whose mother worked at Eaton's many years ago. She told me about the tale of a failed robbery during Christmas within her department.

Evidently, an older woman was working in the ladies' dress register alone. A man wearing an hoodie black came into the register, swung an open knife and demanded the lady to unlock the cash register, and hand the cash. Somehow, the woman's behavior was very different than what most people -- including the robbers-- would imagine.

She turned and said "Young man, where is your mother? Do you know what you're doing this evening? You ought to be embarrassed of yourself. Get out of the way before I notify the police, and they'll have to contact your mother. Now, get out of the way!"

He was shocked by this fierce older woman's refusal to grant him what he wanted , that his eyes widened and he fled, possibly in stupor.

This isn't something I'd recommend trying. It's a great illustration of how frightening someone with a completely unplanned action could be beneficial to you.

#4: Make a plan in advance If an attack happens and you're in the "Black Zone". Your adrenaline level will be that you'll be unable to formulate a sensible plan or come up with an effective escape route. It's the reason it's important to make a plan and to review it prior to time.

For instance, when I'm in the position of protecting a client I study the area in which we'll be ahead of schedule. I am familiar with the terrain, escape routes, the typical crowds and more. I have a variety of plans of escape prior to time should we ever need to make use of them. In my head I practice every possible scenario I can imagine and plan out my plan of action should any of these events occur.

It's not necessary to go into this level of in detail, but it's possible to nevertheless have a strategy in advance of time based on the challenges you're confronted with. For instance, if you live in an area that is rough town, you may want to think about strategies to follow should you be confronted by a robber or a thief.

I know of women who carry pepper spray , or even aerosol hair spray on their hands while wandering around in the rough areas of town. You might want to carry a fake wallet to give to muggers (with some bills and expired debit cards).

It is a good idea to create a plan for the group of what the family should be doing should an incident of break-in happen (for instance, a regular gathering place, a variety of options for exits that children could take and so on.).

Our wife and me have a code word we've agreed to use in the event that either of us are in danger. If she does this while I'm on the phone to her, I'm able to immediately disconnect and contact the police as she's in trouble.

Once you've got your plan practice it over and over in your head. The practice of rehearsing your plan repeatedly over again will enable you to be prepared should you be confronted.

The main point is that in the event that something catastrophic occurs, you'll not be thinking clearly. Your brain will turn back to your animal brain. Therefore, if you practice the plan in advance (even even if just in your mind) it is more likely to recall the plan when you're required to.

"Victorious warriors first win before going to war, whereas defeated warriors start war first and then try to take victory." -" Sun Tzu, The Art of War

#5: Recognize You have Control someone is victimized, they may quickly feel helpless, and even victimized. They lose their feeling of control. When people lose control, despair sets in and they are been truly defeated because it's unlikely to try for escape, or to defend your self.

If you're being attacked It may not be obvious however, you still have some control. You have the option of choosing.

You can choose to either fight or give up. You are able to surrender or attempt to escape. You can choose to observe your attacker and attempt to discover weaknesses or surrender in the hope that someone else will save you. You are able to join them or tell them no.

There is still a degree of control. You have different options. They can be enough to keep you smiling.

Take control of your life in whatever way you can however you can, even if it's by a tiny amount. This will help you keep going forward, instead of falling into a pit of despair. You will be contemplating, trying to outwit your opponent. When you feel you're in control, despair sets in and you decide to give up. Your attacker has already defeated you.

Be aware that your adversaries have not really defeated until you have given up your hope.

Recently, I watched an documentary about the training and training that members of members of the British Special Air Service (SAS) undergoes when they are captured and interrogated by their enemies. One of the lessons they are taught is to keep an element of control.

It could range that is akin to slapping the interrogator behind the back by pointing your tongue at him, pointing the finger, to secretly throwing things off the desk, etc. It is a habit that they are taught to perform these things so that the SAS officer will maintain a certain amount of control and mental stability even in a dangerous situation.

#6: Be aware of the four psychological stages you'll go through If you're attacked, and try to move through them as fast as you can: If someone is attacked, particularly when it's physical and fast-paced, they traverse certain phases of their mental health in their minds as they try to deal with the events happening. In reality, it's an almost predictable process all humans go through.

The most important thing is not to attempt to alter the human mind and alter the process. The most important thing is to be aware about the stages involved and what's about to happen to you , and then work to go through them as swiftly as you can.

Why not get them through in the quickest time possible?

The reason is because the last phases are when you'll have your brainpower and adrenaline working to figure out the best way to fight back and escape. At the beginning of the process, you might be numb and ineffective.

These are four psychological phases that most people experience when they are attacked:

#1: Disorientation "What's taking place to me?"

#2: Denial/Disbelief - "Is this actually taking place to me? I'm not able to believe that it's happening!"

#3: Depression/Questioning - "Why is this happening to me? Do I really want to die? I'm devastated that I'm going to die!"

#4: Displeasure/Anger "I'm annoyed that this has happened to me. Damned if I'm willing allow this to take place in my life!"

This stage is the one you'd like to reach as quickly as you can. It's not always easy for everyone to get there. A few people are trapped in the 3rd phase.

But if you're able to take action, take whatever steps necessary to make it to stage 4 and then take the next steps that you'll have to take to safeguard yourself.

It is important to note that you begin to think and plan at the stage 4 and beyond. In action, you are looking at the situation, considering the best way to respond and identifying weaknesses in your adversaries or opponent, etc.

The fourth stage is also where your survival instincts begin to kick in, in an effort for you to live a better life.

You've probably seen this before , when you've heard stories from other people about how they escaped difficult situations. In the majority of cases they'll tell of an instant of clarity, when they knew exactly what they needed to do to get through the situation.

It's the final step the survival skills are working at full force to help you focus and stay at peace. While you'll remain calm, you'll be able to perform the tasks you must accomplish. You'll be aware and at the high-performance. You'll be able to harness the extraordinary ability to rely on your survival instincts that many times, are detecting subtle and conscious clues connecting them all while telling you how to proceed.

In his amazing work, The Gift of Fear, Gavin DeBecker recounts a tale about one of his customers which shows this in a perfect way. She was assaulted and attacked by a man who been stalking her for several days. She was lying in her bedroom after being assaulted. The man arose and told her to not move. He went to the kitchen. When he returned the man said he'd take her away.

The survival instincts of her started to kick inand she knew --though she was not sure how --that she needed to leave her home and get out of the apartment. She knew with complete conviction that if she continued to stay in the same place as he'd instructed her to, he'd end her life.

As the room was empty she stood up and followed him in a quiet manner, and then left the house when they were working in the kitchen.

She wasn't aware until later the extent to which she was aware that this man was actually likely to murder her if she kept her bedroom. In the future, she recalled the following basic fact: The man shut her bedroom window (which was opened) just moments before telling her not to leave the room.

Her mind was aware of this one small gesture and informed her that he was shutting the window in her bedroom so that no one would be able to hear her screaming. He was determined to kill her. In reality, he been into the kitchen to search for the knife he needed to kill her.

In following her instincts to survive and taking action she had made a difference in her own life.

#7: Don't Blame Youself In this book, I've mentioned that by applying the basic principles of self-defense psychologically to avoid the possibility of avoiding up to 95% attacks. But what happens to the remaining five percent?

What happens when you've tried everything you can but find yourself being assaulted? Don't blame yourself.

Accept that there are occasions when circumstances occur that are outside of your control, and therefore not your blame. There are times when there is nothing one could do differently to avoid being victimized. The fact that you blame yourself will not solve the problem. It is important to accept the reality of the situation as it is and take steps to improve your life. (Remember you're still in the ability to control your situation.)

Make an effort to work through the disbelief, shock and sadness that you experience when you realize you are in this situation and then get to your fear and survival urges which could to save your life. Be sure to trust that they're there. Everyone is one else. They'll be there to help you whenever you require them.

This was illustrated by a courageous young woman who came up to me after my seminar about personal self-protection.

Unfortunately, she been in a rare 5-percent-type of scenario that she couldn't be able to do nothing about. The woman was walking into her apartment at night, when the man appeared out of the blue and held an axe towards her throat. The door was already open. She was forced to let him in and he attacked her.

She let him go as she wanted, after which he gone.

"What would I've done differently in this circumstance?" she asked me. "What was I doing wrong?"

"Absolutely nothing,"" I told you. "You didn't do anything wrong. Actually you did everything right."

"What is your meaning?" she asked.

"You're still alive,"" I declared. "You followed your instincts to survive and did what you had to do in order to be able to survive, however painful that might have been. It's not your fault. You ought to be proud. You're a hero and you made it through."

Her gut instincts informed her that in this scenario she shouldn't be fighting back. Her instincts advised her she'd be able to get through the situation and the likelihood was that he'd go away in the event that she let him do what he wanted to do. Her instincts were right and she'd made it through.

It's clear that this is not the scenario that most people would prefer however, she escaped the worst of circumstances where there was a choice to be raped or murdered and raped. Sometimes, life doesn't offer the best alternatives. She made the best choice she could with the data she had.

Sometimes, there's nothing else to do. Do not blame yourself. Instead, trust your gut instincts, absorb all the information you can, and then do what you must do to stay alive.

Be aware that you'll be able to come out of this. You are more powerful than you realize.

Important Points:

If a fight turns into physical battle, you have ways to combat the situation and stay alive:

Don't let yourself be dragged to a different place.

If you are determined to fight against the attacker, make sure you go to the end and keep going until your attacker can't take you down.

Make use of a distraction to allow yourself the opportunity to escape.

Create a plan in advance of the steps you'll take in case of an attack. Practice it in your head every day.

You will realize that you always have some degree of control over any situation, it will allow you to move ahead.

You should try to go through the four emotional states that affect all people when they are you are attacked. You should get to the final stage as quickly as you can, the phase of anger where you can decide, act and combat the attack.

Don't be a victim. There are times when there is nothing to have changed differently to stop an attack. Accept the situation and think about how you could respond to escape alive.

Do what you can to live - you are more resilient than you realize.

Conclusion

I hope that this book has been helpful to discover the martial art techniques you can apply to protect yourself in the real world. Be aware that these are only the basic ones and there are plenty of other methods you must master in order to protect yourself.

The next step after mastering the strategies described in this book is to search for advice on how you can protect yourself from grapples, holds locks, grapples weapons, as well as fighting with groups of people. These are more complicated areas that will be addressed in other books.